PROSTATE

Diseases & Conditions

2007 Report

Group Director: Gary Strassberg, Belvoir Media Group

Prostate: Diseases & Conditions

Written by Karen Rafinski

Consulting Editor: Eric A. Klein, M.D. Professor of Surgery, Cleveland Clinic Lerner College of Medicine and Section Head, Urologic Oncology, Glickman Urological Institute, Cleveland Clinic, Cleveland, Ohio

Production Editor: Oksana Charla

ISBN: 1-879620-74-X

To order additional copies of this report or for customer service questions, please call 877-300-0253.

TABLE OF CONTENTS
Prostate: Diseases & Conditions

2007
REPORT ON PROSTATE: DISEASES & CONDITIONS

The prostate is a little-understood organ that can cause men a lot of trouble late in life. The organ is intertwined with the male urinary and reproductive systems, often causing debilitating problems in both when it acts up. What are these problems? What should you do about them? This report focuses on providing you with an understanding of prostate conditions, preventive tips, and treatment options.

• • •

HIGHLIGHTS

- Study finds that prostatitis symptoms usually do not worsen over time, but instead stabilize or even improve slightly. (Page 13, Box 2-2)

- Prostate enlargement may not be linked to obesity after all, new research has found. (Page 16, Box 3-2)

- Combination drug therapy works best for men with moderate to large prostates, but does not benefit those with small prostates. (Page 23, Box 3-4)

- Study finds holmium laser enucleation (HoLep), a minimally invasive treatment for prostate enlargement, as effective as traditional surgery. (Page 25, Box 3-7)

- Recent research casts serious doubt on whether saw palmetto benefits men with prostate enlargement. (Page 27, Box 3-9)

- Conflicting studies cast doubt on the value of prostate specific antigen (PSA) screening for prostate cancer. (Page 29, Box 4-1)

- Men who take the drug finasteride to treat prostate enlargement may be more likely to have a prostate cancer detected with a standard PSA screening test. (Page 31, Box 4-2)

- Men with very low PSA levels don't need to be screened every year; every three years is sufficient. (Page 36, Box 4-3)

- Early research finds drinking pomegranate juice may slow the progression of prostate cancer after a recurrence. (Page 40, Box 5-1)

- Studies indicate that prostate cancer may be more dangerous in obese men, who face a greater risk of late detection and recurrence. (Page 41, Box 5-2)

- Delaying surgery and undergoing active surveillance does not raise the incidence of non-curable cancer. (Page 48, Box 6-1)

- Men with prostate cancer tend to rush into treatment and don't consider all the risks of their treatment options. (Page 50, Box 6-2)

- Minimally invasive surgical techniques for prostate cancer reduce recovery time and surgical complications versus traditional open surgery. (Page 52, Box 6-3)

- Review of research on active surveillance raises questions about the best way to monitor men who opt to delay treatment. (Page 60, Box 6-4)

- Hormone therapy may not increase the risk of depression, fatigue and cognitive problems as much as some researchers thought. (Page 62, Box 6-5)

- Combining hormone therapy with vaccine significantly increases its effectiveness in staving off prostate cancer. (Page 64, Box 6-6)

• • •

INTRODUCTION

Women may suffer through childbirth and menopause, but God balanced the scales a bit when he designed the prostate. The bane of middle-aged and older men, this problematic gland can cause a host of debilitating and embarrassing symptoms, from painful urination to sexual problems. Worse, it can turn cancerous and even kill.

Half of all men over age 50 are estimated to have enlarged prostates, and that percentage climbs as they age. Over a lifetime, about one in six men can expect to be diagnosed with prostate cancer. Though the survival rates for this cancer are very high—about 98 percent at five years, according to recent estimates—prostate cancer will kill nearly 30,000 men this year because it is so common.

But despite the threat and the widespread quality-of-life problems caused by the prostate, it remains a little-understood organ. Men facing prostate problems are often frustrated by confusing, even conflicting medical advice. In many cases they must make decisions without the benefit of solid scientific evidence. Researchers don't fully understand how the prostate works, what causes many of the conditions that plague it, or which treatments work best.

Medical debate rages over even the most seemingly simple questions, such as whether it's wise to screen men for prostate cancer. Doctors don't have enough evidence to know which treatments are best for which cancer patients—and there's some evidence that some patients may not benefit from treatment at all. That's a serious problem because prostate cancer treatment can cause onerous side effects, notably impotence and incontinence.

Much research is underway to clarify these issues and others. Frequently, however, patients are left to their own devices in the face of insufficient medical advice. For this reason, if you are facing prostate disease or prostate cancer, you may have to decide on a course of action in the face of alarming ambiguity. This report aims to help you fully understand your options, their risks and benefits, and the latest research so you can make the most informed decision possible. ■

1. ANATOMY OF THE PROSTATE

The prostate is a crucial gland in the male sexual and reproductive system, whose main function is to produce most of the fluid in semen. It is about the size and shape of a walnut and, when healthy, weighs about an ounce. In young boys it is only the size of a pea; when they reach puberty, the prostate undergoes a growth spurt spurred by the surge of hormones. By age 20, it reaches its normal adult size. But typically, it begins growing slowly again, sometimes as early as age 25. It can swell as large as a baseball later in life, causing the urinary symptoms that plague so many older men.

The prostate lies just below the bladder, wrapped around a thin tube called the urethra that delivers urine from the bladder out through the penis (see Box 1-1).

The prostate is composed of glandular tissue and a lot of muscle, divided into three lobes and surrounded by an outer casing. The most important of the gland's products is a liquid protein called prostate specific antigen (PSA).

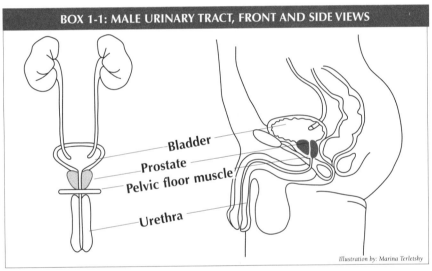

BOX 1-1: MALE URINARY TRACT, FRONT AND SIDE VIEWS

Bladder
Prostate
Pelvic floor muscle
Urethra

Illustration by: Marina Terletshy

Its main function is to liquefy the other thick, jelly-like substances that go into semen, turning it into a thin, milky liquid. That liquid helps deliver sperm outside the body and is crucial to successful natural conception. It may also help energize the sperm and make the vaginal canal a friendlier environment for them.

A tiny bit of PSA is normally secreted into a man's bloodstream, and that is the basis of PSA tests for cancer screening, which will be discussed later.

When a man has an orgasm, muscles squeeze the PSA and other fluid from the prostate into the urethra through tiny pores. There it mixes with fluid from the nearby seminal vesicles, and sperm, which have traveled up from the testicles to form semen. The muscle contractions then force this liquid out during ejaculation. Muscles also close off the bladder so the semen does not mix with urine.

Why the prostate causes so much trouble

Unfortunately, the design of the prostate, wrapped donut-like around the urethra, and nestled so close to key structures in both the urinary and reproductive systems, is the root of many problems. When enlarged or diseased, it squeezes the urethra, blocking the flow of urine. If urine is blocked too long, it can back up into the bladder, which may over-distend and not empty fully. If left untreated, this can permanently damage the bladder. The backed-up urine can also cause urinary tract infections, kidney damage and other complications.

This design also complicates treatment. Because the prostate is intertwined with so many crucial organs, nerves and other important structures, it is difficult to remove or treat without damaging something. Thus, treatment carries a risk of serious side effects like impotence or incontinence.

Symptoms

Many older men simply expect prostate symptoms to be a normal part of aging. They observed their fathers and grandfathers getting up to urinate in the middle of the night so they are not troubled when it happens to them. But ignoring prostate symptoms can cause trouble later on, such as overlooking the early signs of cancer, or letting a treatable condition fester until there is permanent damage. For that reason, consult your doctor if you have any of these symptoms:

- Dribbling urine
- Trouble urinating or even complete loss of ability to urinate
- Frequent urge to urinate
- Burning or painful urination
- Blood in the urine or semen
- Painful ejaculation
- Difficulty having an erection
- Frequent pain in the lower back, hips or upper thighs. ■

2. PROSTATITIS

One of the most common prostate problems is also the most mysterious. Prostatitis is a general term for a painful inflammation of the prostate that can linger on and off for years. It can cause debilitating urinary and sexual symptoms and even destroy fertility. Sometimes it is caused by a simple bacterial infection and can be treated effectively with antibiotics. But in the vast majority of cases, doctors cannot find a source for the inflammation and don't know how to treat it. Yet prostatitis, in all its forms, is estimated to send about two million men each year to the doctor. It's also the one prostate ailment that plagues young and old alike, with men between the ages of 25 and 45 at increased risk.

Because the disease is so common and so poorly understood, the National Institutes of Health (NIH) and other groups have increased research in the area. One problem is that over the years, some doctors have prescribed antibiotics for all forms of prostatitis, regardless of whether there was evidence of an infection. Frustrated by a lack of effective treatments, many men and their doctors have turned to a variety of unproved strategies, from acupuncture to massaging the prostate. Only recently have rigorous scientific studies begun to look at what causes the problem and which treatments work best. But those efforts have not yet established clear results.

Researchers have identified four categories of prostatitis: acute bacterial, chronic bacterial, chronic non-bacterial (also known as chronic pelvic pain syndrome), and acute asymptomatic inflammatory prostatitis. The first two categories do have an effective treatment—antibiotics—but unfortunately account for only a small portion of cases, as low as 10 percent by some estimates.

Acute bacterial prostatitis

This form of prostatitis usually comes on suddenly and is hard to ignore. You may have a fever and chills, other flu-like symptoms, fatigue, pain in the lower abdomen, lower back, or genitals, and a burning sensation when urinating. Other symptoms include difficulty urinating, inability to empty the bladder, and pain with ejaculation or during bowel movements.

If you do experience these symptoms, you should see a doctor immediately. In some rare cases, acute prostatitis can completely block the flow of urine, causing permanent damage to the prostate and urinary system if not treated. A doctor can insert a catheter to drain the bladder until the infection is cured. Also, untreated acute prostatitis can spread infection into the bloodstream, a rare condition that can be life-threatening.

Acute bacterial prostatitis afflicts young and old alike. The infection in the prostate may stem from the same organisms that cause urinary tract infections, such as E. coli, or from some sexually transmitted diseases like gonorrhea or chlamydia.

Risk factors for prostatitis include a recent history of urinary tract infection or sexually transmitted disease or any medical procedures where a catheter was inserted, a habit of starting and stopping during urination, or the practice of unprotected sex, particularly anal sex.

Acute bacterial prostatitis is easy to diagnose because of its relatively sudden onset and systemic symptoms, neither of which are hallmarks of prostate enlargement or cancer.

Once a diagnosis is confirmed, acute prostatitis can be cured with a number of different antibiotics. Your doctor may prescribe a long course of treatment of up to eight weeks to prevent a recurrence that can lead to chronic prostatitis. In rare and severe cases you may have to be hospitalized and given intravenous antibiotics. It's important to follow your doctor's instructions carefully when taking your antibiotics to ensure this doesn't happen. When you have finished treatment you should return to the doctor and be tested to be sure that the infection is gone.

Chronic bacterial prostatitis

This form of prostatitis develops more slowly and is usually less severe than the acute form, but it's far harder to cure and can last for years. The symptoms are similar to the acute form, but the problem may come and go or appear to be getting better at times, only to worsen. Symptoms include a slight fever, recurrent bladder infections, painful ejaculation or urination, pain in the lower abdomen, lower back or genitals, frequent nighttime urination, difficulty urinating or occasional blood in the semen or urine.

Sometimes chronic prostatitis is caused by bacteria that are left behind after acute prostatitis or a urinary tract infection. But many times there has been no acute infection and the cause of the problem isn't clear. Bacteria may infect the prostate after being introduced by a catheter during a medical procedure or during an injury to the urinary system. Or bacteria may have drifted there from an infection elsewhere in the body. Risk factors for chronic bacterial prostatitis are the same as for acute prostatitis, and diagnosis and treatment is also similar. Your doctor will prescribe antibiotics, though he is likely to prescribe a long course of up to 12 weeks or more. Chronic infections are often harder to cure than the acute type and sometimes are never fully eliminated. In those cases, a low-dose antibiotic may be prescribed permanently to keep the problem under control. Because this infection is so difficult to treat you should follow your doctor's directions about taking your antibiotics scrupulously and be sure to return when you're done so you can be tested to confirm the bacteria has cleared your system. Otherwise, the condition may return (see Box 2-1).

> ### Box 2-1: Preventing prostatitis
>
> Many cases of prostatitis are not preventable. But you can reduce your risk by:
>
> - Practicing safe sex
>
> - Washing your hands after bowel movements and before touching your penis to prevent transferring bacteria
>
> - Following your doctor's directions carefully when taking antibiotics for acute prostatitis or a urinary tract infection
>
> - Urinating in a steady stream without starting and stopping

Chronic non-bacterial prostatitis

Unfortunately, most men with chronic prostatitis suffer from the more mysterious and still more difficult to treat non-bacterial form. Also known as chronic prostatitis/chronic pelvic pain syndrome or CP/CPPS, this form of prostatitis is an inflammation of the prostate with no known cause. It produces about the same symptoms as chronic bacterial prostatitis, except that it usually doesn't cause a fever. The biggest difference is that your doctor won't detect any signs of bacteria when he does the standard tests on urine and fluid from your prostate.

But even then, things are rarely clear-cut with this enigmatic disease. Sometimes doctors will find white blood cells in your urine and semen, evidence that the immune system is rallying to fight some sort of infection, even though there's no evidence of an actual infection. It's also possible to have a form of CP/CPPS that doesn't produce symptoms at all—luckily enough—and requires no treatment. This asymptomatic form is sometimes picked up during routine exams or when doctors test for fertility problems.

The causes of CP/CPPS remain shrouded in mystery, but some new and more promising ideas are now under study. Some think that it may simply be an undetected infection, based on evidence that more careful and longer culturing picks up bacterial infections missed in early tests. Or the cause could be some unknown infectious agent that isn't showing up on the available tests. Another camp believes that it may be an auto-immune reaction in the prostate, in which the body attacks itself in the same way it would mount a defense against a bacterial infection. Other theories blame tension in muscles near the prostate, or abnormalities in the urinary system.

It's important to remember that at this time, all of this remains theory and not fact. More research is needed to pinpoint a cause. Many researchers also think that several of these factors, or other unknown causes, may cause different forms of the problem or combine to create the condition. Unfortunately, this enigma makes treatment decisions difficult.

Acute asymptomatic inflammatory prostatitis

This occurs when a man has no symptoms of prostatitis, such as pain, but when he has signs of infection-fighting cells in his semen. It's usually discovered inadvertently when doctors are performing tests for other conditions such as infertility or prostate cancer. It does not require treatment.

Treatment

Because of this uncertainty, doctors work to control symptoms, rather than strive for a cure. Very often, doctors will start with a round of antibiotics, on the assumption that the cause is an undetected infection. But there is serious debate about this issue. Some researchers oppose the practice because they say it's not effective and exposes men to unnecessary side effects from the antibiotics. Research on the issue is scant, but so far has failed to prove that there's any real benefit to taking antibiotics when there's no evidence of a bacterial infection.

Two drugs normally used to treat prostate enlargement, finasteride (Proscar) and tamsulosin (Flomax), have received attention because some early studies indicated they improved symptoms. However, more rigorous trials are needed to determine whether there really is a benefit to them because the evidence so far is mixed. One trial found that neither antibiotics nor tamsulosin had any significant benefits. The October 2004 study, published in the *Annals of Internal Medicine*, looked at 196 men with chronic prostatitis/chronic pelvic pain syndrome who had moderate symptoms for an average of 6.2 years. They either were given the antibiotic ciprofloxacin (Cipro) or tamsulosin (Flomax), a combination of both drugs, or a placebo. After six weeks of treatment, none of these groups reported any significant improvement in their symptoms. Previous research has also failed to find a benefit for the use of antibiotics to treat CP/CPPS. But two previous, though smaller, trials had shown a benefit to drugs like tamsulosin when used for up to six months. More research is needed to determine whether there truly is a benefit.

Also, over-the-counter pain relievers such as ibuprofen or aspirin seem to reduce pain for some patients. Just be aware that these medications, with prolonged use, can cause ulcers and intestinal bleeding.

Unfortunately, in the absence of a cure and because current treatments don't work for all patients, many men go through years of trial and error to find a way to reduce their symptoms. It's important as you do this to keep in close contact with your doctor, who can help you through the process.

Though this process can be frustrating, it's not completely hopeless. A new study has found that most men's prostatitis symptoms don't usually worsen over time, and about a third of the men in the study reported improvement in their symptoms over a two-year period (see Box 2-2).

There are also some things you can do on your own that sometimes help alleviate symptoms. Warm baths may alleviate low-back pain. So can special exercises that stretch and relax the pelvis and lower back, which you can learn from a physical therapist. Some men have reported relief from biofeedback, which teaches you how to relax certain muscles and control other bodily responses. Others find acupuncture helpful. These last two methods have some support from research, but the studies were not rigorous enough to be considered solid evidence. Some men have tried alternative treatments such as saw palmetto and bee pollen, but there's little scientific evidence so far that they work. One recent study found no benefit to taking saw palmetto.

Some doctors and patients say that making lifestyle changes can help reduce symptoms, though these methods haven't been studied to see

---

NEW FINDING

Box 2-2: Prostatitis symptoms stabilize or improve over time

A new study has found that prostatitis symptoms do not usually worsen over the long run but rather stabilize.

The research, published in the *Journal of Urology's* February 2006 issue, followed 293 men with Chronic Prostatitis/Chronic Pelvic Pain Syndrome, for two years and evaluated their symptoms and quality of life with a standard questionnaire.

After two years, 31 percent of the men reported significantly improved symptoms and the average improvement was 5 points on the 43-point NIH standard scale. Most of the improvement occurred in the first three months of follow-up during the study. Though some men reported ups and downs, there was no evidence that their overall condition declined over time.

if they work. Drinking extra fluids, eliminating alcohol and caffeine, cutting back on spicy foods and urinating frequently may be helpful.

Complications

There is no evidence that prostatitis increases your risk of cancer—but some researchers are studying the issue to see if the inflammation it causes might play a role in cancer risk. Be aware, however, that prostatitis can affect the PSA screening test for prostate cancer. The condition may cause an increase in the amount of PSA in your blood, which can be a sign of cancer but is not necessarily so. For this reason, your doctor should take a new PSA test after you've been treated with antibiotics and should take your prostatitis into account when screening you for cancer.

Also, prostatitis can interfere with the development of semen and ejaculation and therefore cause fertility problems. Some studies have shown that men with the condition have poor sperm quality, which can also affect fertility. ■

3. PROSTATE ENLARGEMENT

Here's an unpleasant reward at the end of a long life: sooner or later, nearly all men will have to contend with the vexing urinary problems caused by an enlarged prostate. More than half of men in their 60s suffer some symptoms and the percentage increases as men age. About 90 percent or more of men in their 70s and 80s have the problem. Prostate enlargement, also known as benign prostatic hyperplasia or BPH, sent eight million men to their doctor in the year 2000, according to the NIH.

Prostate enlargement has its roots in the slow growth of the prostate that is normal throughout a man's life. Over time, it can progress from the size of a walnut to as large as a peach. This growth rarely causes any symptoms before a man hits the age of 45. But sometime in middle or old age, symptoms begin to appear. The trouble starts when the prostate begins to swell inward, choking off the urethra (see boxes 3-1A and 3-1B). This blockage begins to damage and irritate the bladder, which may begin to contract even when only a little urine is present. This is what causes older men to feel the need to urinate more often. Eventually, the bladder may weaken and no longer be able to empty completely.

No one is quite sure what causes the prostate to enlarge, but it seems the growth may be regulated by normal male hormones such as testosterone. Men who are castrated before puberty do not suffer prostate enlargement; neither do men who are unable to produce a hormone called dihydrotestosterone (DHT). But exactly how hormonal

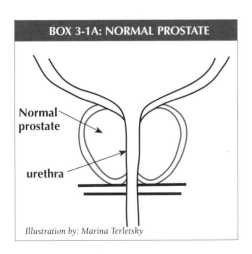

BOX 3-1A: NORMAL PROSTATE

Normal prostate

urethra

Illustration by: Marina Terletsky

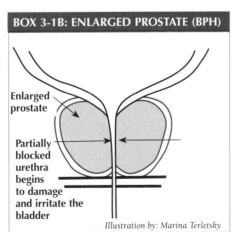

BOX 3-1B: ENLARGED PROSTATE (BPH)

Enlarged prostate

Partially blocked urethra begins to damage and irritate the bladder

Illustration by: Marina Terletsky

changes may cause the prostate to enlarge as men age remains a mystery.

Because the problem is far more common in the United States and Europe than it is in other parts of the world, particularly Asia, some have speculated that diet may play a role. One study in the *Journal of Clinical Nutrition* found that men who consumed more calories and protein had a modestly higher risk of prostate enlargement, as did those who consumed quantities of certain fats. But the theory is not proven and needs more research. Researchers also have speculated that obesity might be related to prostate enlargement, but a new study has cast serious doubt on that link (see Box 3-2).

Recent research has looked at a potential but unproved link between high blood pressure and prostate enlargement—two conditions that may have similar causes. Married men are more likely to suffer the problem than single men, again, for unknown reasons.

Symptoms

What is known is that as men continue to live longer, the incidence of prostate enlargement continues to increase. They suffer a range of symptoms that include:

- Weak urine stream
- Increased urgency of urination
- Dribbling or leaking
- Frequent need to urinate, especially at night
- Difficulty starting to urinate
- Starting and stopping while urinating
- Inability to empty the bladder
- Blood in the urine
- Urinary tract infection

Many men experience just a few of these symptoms, or such mild symptoms that they are not bothered by the condition. Only about half ever seek medical treatment for the problem. However, doctors advise that you have a check-up if you experience any of these symptoms to be sure they are not caused by cancer.

The amount and severity of symptoms you may experience has nothing to do with the actual size of your prostate. Some men with relatively small prostates experience severe problems, while others with large prostates have few symptoms. Also, in many men symptoms do not get worse over time even though the prostate continues to grow. Sometimes symptoms improve on their own, for reasons that aren't fully understood.

Occasionally, symptoms worsen suddenly, and a man completely loses his ability to urinate, an emergency condition that requires immediate medical attention to relieve pain and prevent the bladder from rupturing. Often this problem, called acute urinary retention, can be triggered by over-the-counter cold and allergy medications which contain decongestants. A potential side effect of these medications can prevent the bladder from opening and emptying its urine. If your prostate is enlarged, the problem can also be triggered by alcohol, cold weather, and inactivity.

Recent research indicates that common prescription painkillers may also increase your risk. Non-steroidal anti-inflammatory drugs, or NSAIDs, may double the risk of acute urinary retention, a recent study found. NSAIDs include many common prescription drugs such as celecoxib (Celebrex), ibuprofen (Motrin and Advil), naproxen (Anaprox) and many others. Many are also sold over-the-counter, though the study did not look at those products. The July 2005 study, published in the *Archives of Internal Medicine*, looked at 536 patients with acute urinary retention and compared them to more than 5,000 men with similar medical histories who did not develop acute urinary retention. Researchers found that men who were taking prescription NSAIDs had twice the risk of acute urinary retention as men who didn't. Those who'd recently started taking the drugs were at the highest risk, as were those who were taking the maximum recommended daily dosage or more of the drugs. More research is needed to confirm the link.

Chronic retention of urine due to an enlarged prostate can cause permanent bladder and kidney damage, bladder stones, and recurrent urinary tract infections.

Testing and diagnosis

If you have symptoms of prostate enlargement, your doctor may refer you to a urologist, a specialist who deals with urinary and sexual problems in men. You will be given a number of tests to rule out cancer and other conditions. The specific tests will vary depending on your doctor's concerns.

Most likely, your doctor will start with a physical exam, during which he will insert a gloved finger into your rectum so that he can feel the part of the prostate that lies nearby (see box 3-3). This will tell him if your prostate is enlarged and can give him hints about whether the problem is due to cancer, prostatitis, or some other cause.

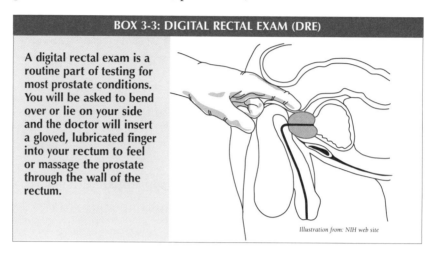

BOX 3-3: DIGITAL RECTAL EXAM (DRE)

A digital rectal exam is a routine part of testing for most prostate conditions. You will be asked to bend over or lie on your side and the doctor will insert a gloved, lubricated finger into your rectum to feel or massage the prostate through the wall of the rectum.

Illustration from: NIH web site

To rule out cancer, he may also recommend a PSA blood test. The difficulty here is that the PSA readings can be hard to interpret. Prostate enlargement can cause your PSA levels to rise in the absence of cancer. This test may give your doctor a broad guideline about how to proceed, but be aware it cannot tell you for sure if you do or do not have cancer. The ins and outs of PSA testing are covered in chapter 4.

Your doctor is also likely to give you the following questionnaire, called the American Urological Association Score, about your urinary symptoms to help assess the severity of the problem. Circle where appropriate.

Incomplete emptying: Over the past month, how often have you had a sensation of not emptying your bladder completely after you finished urinating?

Not at all	Less than 1 time in 5	Less than half the time	About half the time	More than half the time	Almost Always	Your Score
0	1	2	3	4	5	_____

Frequency: Over the past month, how often have you had to urinate again less than 2 hours after you finished urinating?

Not at all	Less than 1 time in 5	Less than half the time	About half the time	More than half the time	Almost Always	Your Score
0	1	2	3	4	5	_____

Intermittency: Over the past month, how often have you found that you stopped and started again several times when you urinated?

Not at all	Less than 1 time in 5	Less than half the time	About half the time	More than half the time	Almost Always	Your Score
0	1	2	3	4	5	_____

Urgency: Over the past month, how often have you found it difficult to postpone urination?

Not at all	Less than 1 time in 5	Less than half the time	About half the time	More than half the time	Almost Always	Your Score
0	1	2	3	4	5	_____

Weak stream: Over the past month, how often have you had a weak stream?

Not at all	Less than 1 time in 5	Less than half the time	About half the time	More than half the time	Almost Always	Your Score
0	1	2	3	4	5	_____

Straining: Over the past month, how often have you had to push or strain to begin urination?

Not at all	Less than 1 time in 5	Less than half the time	About half the time	More than half the time	Almost Always	Your Score
0	1	2	3	4	5	_____

Nocturia: Over the past month or so, how often did you get up to urinate from the time you went to bed until the time you got up in the morning?

Not at all	Less than 1 time in 5	Less than half the time	About half the time	More than half the time	Almost Always	Your Score
0	1	2	3	4	5	_____

Add up your scores for total AUA score = _____

Quality of life due to urinary symptoms: If you were to spend the rest of your life with your urinary condition just the way it is now, how would you feel about that?

Delighted	Pleased	Mostly satisfied	Mixed	Mostly dissatisfied	Unhappy	Terrible

Score	Severity
0 to 7	Mild
8 to 19	Moderate
20 to 35	Severe

If your doctor suspects BPH, he may want to do a few other tests that can help him assess the severity of the problem and how best to treat it. These include:

- **A urinary flow test** that requires you to urinate into a device that measures the amount of urine. A peak flow rate of 15 milliliters per second or above is normal; anything less than 10 indicates a problem that may require treatment.

- **An ultrasound** test or insertion of a catheter to check if you can fully empty your bladder.

- **A special X-ray** called an intravenous urogram or an ultrasound that can help your doctor assess the size of your prostate and how badly it's obstructing the urethra.

- **A cytoscopy,** a procedure in which your doctor inserts a tiny lens and light into the urethra so he can see the extent of the blockage.

Treatment

New drugs and less-invasive surgical procedures have steadily improved the treatment options available to men with prostate enlargement and greatly reduced the unpleasant side effects. Some doctors advocate early treatment of even mild symptoms because it can reduce your risk of complications, such as infection, bleeding, bladder and kidney damage. But these problems are rare, particularly if your doctor is monitoring your condition. Plus, some studies have shown that the symptoms will clear up on their own in about one-third of mild cases. Up to half of men with mild symptoms will not experience any worsening of the condition. The rest will experience a gradual worsening and may ultimately require treatment. Your doctor may suggest that you do nothing at all if your symptoms are mild except undergo a period of "active surveillance." This means you will return to the doctor for regular checkups so he can assess whether your condition is worsening and order treatment before serious complications arise.

In the meantime, there are some simple lifestyle changes that can help you reduce the symptoms of prostate enlargement and prevent them from worsening. You might want to:

- Stop drinking after 7 p.m. to reduce the need to urinate during the night.
- Reduce alcohol and caffeine, especially at night, because they increase urine production.
- Completely empty the bladder whenever you urinate.
- Avoid decongestants, which can lead to urinary retention.
- Exercise. Moderate exercise seems to reduce urinary symptoms.

However, if your symptoms worsen to the point where you are uncomfortable or they are eroding your quality of life, treatment can help. If you are having trouble emptying your bladder, treatment may become necessary to prevent bladder and kidney damage.

Because some of the drugs and surgical procedures used to treat BPH are relatively new, researchers haven't yet established which work best for different patients and which are safest. However, the National Institutes of Health is conducting a clinical trial comparing drug therapy to several minimally invasive procedures in hopes of sorting out which options are best. Those results should come due in the next few years.

Drugs

Medication has become the most common treatment for prostate enlargement and is usually the first line of defense. There are two classes of FDA-approved drugs for this condition. The first class, known as 5-alpha-reductase inhibitors, work by blocking the hormone DHT that causes the prostate to grow. These drugs, finasteride (Proscar or Propecia) and dutasteride (Avodart) shrink the prostate in most men. For some men with larger prostates or serious symptoms, these drugs reduce symptoms and appear to also prevent the condition from progressing, thus preventing or delaying the need for invasive treatment. But they tend to be less effective for those with smaller prostates.

A study suggested that finasteride may reduce the overall risk of prostate cancer by about 25 percent, but it may cause a small increase in the chance of getting an aggressive cancer that is far more deadly than the low-grade cancers it appears to prevent. The study focused on healthy men with PSA levels under 3, normal digital rectal exams and AUA symptoms scores less than 20. More research is needed to determine the real risk of the drug. You may want to talk to your doctor about your personal risks and concerns about prostate cancer if you are considering treatment with finasteride. Side effects are usually minimal, but a small percentage of men will experience breast tenderness or swelling, impotence, decreased libido, and reduced semen volume during ejaculation. It can also take a long time to work. You may not notice any improvement for three to six months. The drug also can lower your PSA levels, affecting the interpretation of your prostate cancer screening test. One recent study has found that finasteride may actually make the PSA test more sensitive and may lead to better detection of prostate cancer at all stages. Dutasteride has been shown in at least one clinical trial to be slightly more effective than finasteride and is considered a viable alternative to finasteride. It has the same side effects.

Prostate enlargement is also treated with alpha-blockers, originally developed to treat high blood pressure but also effective in reducing prostate symptoms. They work by relaxing the muscles around the bladder's opening to the urethra, making it easier to urinate. There are four FDA approved alpha-blockers for this use: terazosin (Hytrin), doxazosin (Cardura), and two specifically designed for prostate treatment, tamsulosin, (Flomax) and alfuzosin (Uroxatral). These drugs work for most men and take effect within a few days. Side effects for some men can include impotence, headaches, dizziness, fatigue, and sometimes low blood pressure. The drugs are equally effective, but tamsulosin or alfuzosin cause fewer systemic side effects. To avoid side effects, your doctor may need to adjust the dose or start you on a low dose and gradually increase it. However, unlike finasteride, the alpha-blockers do not shrink the prostate or appear to stop the progression of the problem.

You should also know that tamsulosin may increase your risk of complications during cataract surgery. An April 2005 study published in the *Journal of Cataract and Refractive Surgery* found that tamsulosin (Flomax) appeared to cause the pupil to contract and the iris to move. These problems can cause complications during surgery, including rupture of the part of the natural lens of the eye that remains after surgery. The study looked at 900 cataract surgeries and found that 2.2 percent of patients were affected by the problem. Of those patients affected by the problem, 94 percent had taken tamsulosin. More research is needed to confirm whether there really is a problem, but the study authors suggest that men who are undergoing cataract surgery be taken off the drug for a few weeks before surgery to minimize the risk.

Until recently, most doctors started prostate enlargement patients on an alpha-blocker alone since the drug rapidly relieves symptoms and usually produces few side effects. But recent research is causing some doctors to rethink the issue. A long-term study found that treating patients with both finasteride and an alpha-blocker boosted the effectiveness of either drug alone, reducing symptoms by about two-thirds. It also reduced the risk of the disease progressing and needing surgical or other invasive treatment by about two-thirds. However, some researchers are sounding a note of caution because the cancer risks of finasteride are not yet fully understood and because most men with enlarged prostates do fine on just an alpha-blocker and never see their problem worsen. In fact, 83 percent of study participants on a placebo did not have their condition worsen—so some researchers argue there is no need for combination therapy for most men. The study found that men with high PSA levels or particularly large prostates were most likely to need surgery eventually and therefore most likely to benefit from the two-drug therapy at the onset. A new study has also confirmed the finding that men with larger prostates do better on combination therapy, while men with relatively small prostates don't seem to benefit from the combination approach (see Box 3-4).

Those whose condition worsens while on an alpha-blocker may also benefit from treatment with both drugs. One commonly used strategy is to begin with combination therapy to get the immediate symptom relief from the alpha-blocker while waiting for the 5-alpha-reductase inhibitor to shrink the prostate over three to six months, followed by stopping the alpha-blocker to save on cost and side effects. Be aware though that both drugs lower blood pressure and some of the 5-alpha-reductase inhibitors are not meant to be combined with other blood-pressure-lowering drugs.

Non-surgical treatment

Unfortunately, medications don't work for all men. Over the years, researchers have developed a number of treatments that are less invasive than surgery for these patients. These procedures work better than medication, but they may not always be as effective as surgery in eliminating symptoms. Some of them don't have a long history so their long-term benefits and side effects haven't been fully studied. But unlike surgery, they don't require a lengthy hospital stay, and recovery is typically easier.

Usually these therapies use heat to destroy a portion of the enlarged prostate. The most common is transurethral microwave therapy, or TUMT, which uses the heat from microwaves to destroy some of the prostate tissue around the urethra, eliminating the blockage (see Box 3-5). During the procedure, a catheter with a microwave antenna at the tip is inserted into the urethra, and allowed to heat the tissue. Cool water circulates around the antenna to protect the urethra, but the prostate tissue surrounding it is destroyed, opening up a passage for urine to travel through freely. The one-hour procedure is done under local anesthesia. You may feel some heat, spasms, or have a strong desire to urinate. Most men can return home the same day of the

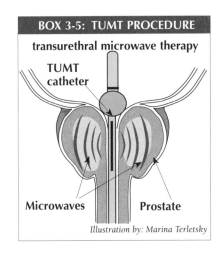

BOX 3-5: TUMT PROCEDURE

transurethral microwave therapy

TUMT catheter

Microwaves   Prostate

Illustration by: Marina Terletsky

Box 3-6: TUMT vs. surgery

Box 3-6: TUMT vs. surgery

Surgery seems to do a better job of relieving the symptoms of prostate enlargement than transurethral microwave therapy (TUMT) over the long haul, though the minimally invasive procedure is an effective short-term treatment, according to a review of research on the issue. The review, published in the *British Journal of Urology*, looked at six studies involving 540 patients. Taken together, the men who had TUMT saw their score on a standard symptom survey decrease 65 percent, compared to 77 percent for men who had surgery. The men who had surgery suffered more side effects, including retrograde ejaculation, than men who had TUMT. But men who underwent a TUMT procedure were more likely to need subsequent treatment because their prostate enlargement symptoms returned.

procedure, but you may have to wear a catheter for several days until you heal enough to urinate normally.

The procedure works well for 60 to 70 percent of patients, at least initially, and they should see a reduction in symptoms. It will not help those who can no longer empty their bladder and seems to work best for those who have mild to moderate enlargement of the prostate. Also, research indicates that while TUMT causes fewer side effects than surgery, many men will experience a return of symptoms over the years and may require additional treatment (see Box 3-6). More research on long-term effectiveness is needed.

It may take several weeks for symptoms to clear up. Side effects include a reduction in the amount of semen you produce. There is a low risk of impotence and incontinence. TUMT carries a lower risk of retrograde ejaculation (also referred to as dry climax), a condition that causes infertility, than surgery. In retrograde ejaculation, semen flows back into the bladder instead of out through the penis during orgasm. This is normally prevented by a muscle that blocks the entrance to the bladder during orgasm, but prostate surgery may cut this muscle, allowing the semen into the bladder. However, this is harmless.

Another version of this kind of heat therapy is called transurethral needle ablation (TUNA). In this case, a catheter is inserted with two needles that send out a low-level radio signal to core the prostate in the same manner as TUMT. As with TUMT, this procedure is not effective for those with very large prostates. Patients who underwent a TUNA procedure maintained an improvement in their symptoms for at least five years, according to a study published in the June 2004 issue of the *Journal of Urology*. The study looked at 121 men with prostate enlargement who were assigned to either surgery or a TUNA procedure. Both groups saw their symptoms improve and maintained their improvement for five years. However, the surgery group had more side effects including retrograde ejaculation, impotence, and incontinence. Larger studies with longer-term follow-up are still needed to determine the long-term effectiveness of TUNA. Side effects include urine retention, blood in your urine, painful urination and a small risk of retrograde ejaculation.

Recent research has produced promising results for a laser treatment called holmium laser enucleation of the prostate, or HoLep (see

Box 3-7). HoLep uses a laser to destroy excess prostate tissue in a manner similar to other heat therapies, by threading a tiny laser into the urethra to destroy excess prostate tissue. The procedure usually causes little bleeding and recovery time is reduced. Unlike some other minimally invasive procedures, it can be used on men with large prostates. It also seems to cause fewer side effects such as impotence or incontinence. However, there is not a lot of large-scale, long-term research on this procedure, so it's not yet known if these results will hold up in the long run.

One new option involves using a high-powered laser to vaporize the enlarged tissues of the prostate to relieve symptoms. Called photoselective vaporization of the prostate, or PVP, this outpatient procedure removes prostate tissue with minimal blood loss. Most patients are able to resume normal activities in a few days. There is a risk of increased urinary urgency and frequency, but this problem usually clears up quickly. Early research indicates that PVP works as well as a minimally invasive surgical procedure called transurethral resection of the prostate, or TURP, and may cause fewer side effects. But more long-term studies are needed to confirm these results and to determine whether the benefit of PVP will be long-lasting.

Surgery

Surgery used to be the most common treatment for an enlarged prostate, but its use has declined in recent years, thanks to the advent of effective medications and less-invasive procedures. However, it is still the most effective method to relieve symptoms, with the best track record long-term. It may be necessary for some men with very large prostates, severe symptoms or those who have complicating factors like frequent urinary tract infections or kidney or bladder problems.

Unlike prostate cancer surgery, in surgery for prostate enlargement much of the prostate is left behind. Typically, only the enlarged tissue inside the prostate that is squeezing the urethra shut is removed, leaving the outer portion behind. This reduces the side effects and complications compared to prostate cancer surgery, but it does not completely eliminate the risk of impotence and incontinence.

About 90 percent of all surgery for benign prostate enlargement is done with a minimally invasive procedure called transurethral resection of the prostate, or TURP (see Box 3-8). Because there is no open incision, the procedure is far less traumatic and heals more quickly than open surgery. An instrument called a resectoscope, which contains a light and an electrical loop for both cutting tissue and sealing blood vessels, is inserted into the penis. The surgeon uses the wire loop to hollow out the enlarged tissue that is blocking the urethra. Irrigation fluid is used to flush the tissue out of the body at the end of the operation.

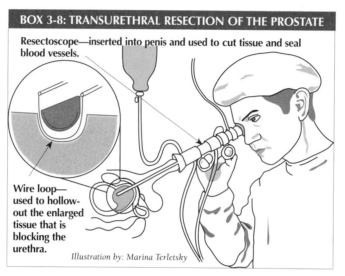

BOX 3-8: TRANSURETHRAL RESECTION OF THE PROSTATE

Resectoscope—inserted into penis and used to cut tissue and seal blood vessels.

Wire loop—used to hollow-out the enlarged tissue that is blocking the urethra.

Illustration by: Marina Terletsky

The procedure takes about 90 minutes and requires a short hospital stay of one to three days. You will probably have to use a catheter for a few days.

TURP usually relieves urinary symptoms within a few days. You may experience some pain at first when urinating. The procedure may cause impotence and/or incontinence, but these problems are usually temporary. Special exercises can help restore bladder control; and sexual function usually is not affected other than retrograde ejaculation.

In some cases, when a man has an extremely large prostate, bladder damage, or other complications, an old-fashioned open surgery must be performed. In this procedure the surgeon makes an incision in the abdomen to reach the prostate and then scoops out the inside to take the pressure off the bladder. This is the safest bet for those with very large prostates, but it can carry more risks than TURP since it requires open surgery. However, the risk of permanent incontinence or impotence is very low. The procedure also is sometimes used when damage to the bladder or other structures needs to be repaired as well. It usually requires a three- to five-day hospital stay, and a catheter may have to be worn for a few days.

With all surgery you can expect to see some blood in your urine for a while. This is normal and shouldn't alarm you unless you develop blood clots. You should notice that urinating becomes easier and less frequent as you heal. Surgery for prostate enlargement doesn't often cause a loss of potency, but it cannot restore potency if it was lost before the operation. Some men may notice that they no longer produce semen when they have an orgasm. This condition, described earlier, is called retrograde ejaculation or dry climax. Although it is not a health risk—the semen, which flows into the bladder instead of out of the penis, will be flushed out when urinating—it will prevent fathering a child in the usual fashion. This can be hard to get used to; however, it should not affect the quality of sexual climax.

After you have healed from surgery, it is still necessary to see your doctor for routine prostate checks. Prostate surgery leaves behind a lot of prostate tissue so it does not reduce your risk of cancer. Also, because the tissue can continue to grow, you may eventually experience symptoms again. However, this usually only affects men who have surgery at a young age, as the surgery usually holds off symptoms for at least 15 years. Only about 10 percent of men with prostate enlargement ever need a second surgery.

Sometimes scar tissue from the surgery causes additional problems that need treatment. It can block the opening to the bladder or narrow the urethra, causing urinary problems similar to those caused by prostate enlargement. This can be treated by your doctor with a simple surgical procedure or by stretching the urethra.

Alternatives

You may have seen a variety of alternative herbal products advertised as cures for benign prostate enlargement, but you should be skeptical of most of them. Most have not been studied in rigorous scientific fashion, and their claims are often based on dubious science.

The most popular is saw palmetto, which has undergone numerous clinical trials that seemed to indicate that it worked. But a new study has cast serious doubt on that (see Box 3-9). The research, published in the *New England Journal of Medicine* in February 2006, found no evidence of a benefit to taking a specific preparation of saw palmetto twice a day for a year.

This directly contradicts a previous review of medical literature on saw palmetto that did find a benefit. In 1998, an analysis published in the *Journal of the American Medical Association*, looked at about 18 studies and determined that saw palmetto did work. It found that the herb was about as effective as the drug finasteride in reducing

NEW FINDING
Box 3-9: Doubt cast on the value of saw palmetto

A recent study found that saw palmetto performed no better than a sugar pill in relieving the symptoms of prostate enlargement.

The study, published in the *New England Journal of Medicine* in February 2006, looked at 225 men over age 49 who had moderate to severe symptoms of prostate enlargement. The men were given a placebo or a twice-daily dose of 160 milligrams of saw palmetto and followed for a year.

The men given saw palmetto did no better than those who weren't in terms of their symptom scores on the standard American Urological Association survey, urinary flow rate, prostate size or PSA levels. That remained true even when researchers considered how large the men's prostates were and how severe their symptoms before treatment.

Because this was a double-blinded, placebo-controlled study—the gold standard of clinical trials and a superior format to most previous trials of saw palmetto—it casts serious doubt on the value of saw palmetto. However, researchers said there was one limitation to the study in that it only tested a single preparation and dose of saw palmetto, so it's theoretically possible that a different dosage or preparation might work. But there's no evidence of what that preparation or dose would be.

symptoms but had fewer side effects. But it's important to know that there are limitations on this kind of analysis, which depends on comparing many studies conducted with different methods and not always the highest scientific standards. Most of the studies were short-term and therefore could not determine if saw palmetto would work over the long-term. The best way to determine if saw palmetto really works and is safe long-term is through a clinical trial. The NIH is currently conducting such a trial, but those results are not yet in.

Also, herbal products in the U.S. are not regulated by the Food and Drug Administration (FDA) and therefore you have no guarantee that the product you buy really contains saw palmetto, or that it hasn't been contaminated with other products that could affect its potency and safety.

You should know that at least one study of over-the-counter supplements sold for men with prostate conditions found that they rarely delivered what the label promised. The study, published in the *Journal of Urology*, found that half of the six saw palmetto supplements actually contained less than 20 percent of the dose promised on the label when they were tested in a lab. One product contained only three percent of the amount of saw palmetto it was supposed to contain. Still others had more than the recommended dose. ■

4. DECIDING WHETHER PROSTATE CANCER SCREENING IS RIGHT FOR YOU

Sooner or later, all men have to face a decision about whether to be screened for prostate cancer. This may seem like a no-brainer, since the PSA test is often billed as a simple blood test that can detect cancer early and save your life. But it's actually quite a bit more complicated than that. The medical community is deeply split on the issue since there is little strong evidence to date that the PSA test really does save lives (see Box 4-1). Opponents of the test argue that without a clear-cut benefit, screening isn't worth the risk because treatment carries

NEW FINDING
Box 4-1: Conflicting results on the benefit of PSA screening

As so often happens with prostate cancer screening, two recent studies gave conflicting reports on the value of PSA screening. One study that compared men who had been given PSA tests with those who weren't found that there was no benefit to screening in terms of extending lives. Another study found that there was a benefit.

One study, published in January 2006 in the *Archives of Internal Medicine*, looked at 501 men who died after being diagnosed with prostate cancer. They were compared to men with similar characteristics who were not diagnosed with prostate cancer.

The study found about equal rates of screening among both groups of men. About 14 percent of prostate cancer patients had been screened and about 14 percent of those without the disease had been screened.

Researchers could find no benefit to being screened even when they looked only at those men who died specifically of prostate cancer as opposed to other causes. The men who had been screened did not live longer than those who weren't.

There are some serious limitations to the study. The population studied was older—about half over 70—and many researchers believe that older men may not benefit from PSA testing. Also, researchers only looked at an eight-year period in the 1990s, which may not have been long enough to detect the benefits of screening.

Another study, published in the *Journal of Urology* in August 2005, worked in a similar way. It compared 236 men with prostate cancer that had spread through the body to 462 healthy patients with similar characteristics. It found that men with prostate cancer were about half as likely to have been screened for the disease as men without if they were between 45 and 59, and about two-thirds as likely to have been screened if they were between 60 and 84 years old. This suggests that screening may reduce the risk of prostate cancer spreading.

Neither of these studies provides the last word on the subject, which will have to be settled by randomized clinical trials. Two are underway in the U.S. and Europe but the results are not expected until 2009.

a risk of serious side effects such as impotence and incontinence.

One leading proponent of prostate cancer screening, Thomas A. Stamey, MD, of Stanford University, has changed his opinion, warning that the PSA test is no longer useful. In a study in the Journal of Urology, he found the test was picking up too many harmless slow-growing cancers and causing many unnecessary prostate surgeries. The issue is further complicated by research that indicates the screening test does pick up prostate cancer before it spreads, but also that the test misses many aggressive cancers. And recent research hints that it may be more important to look at how fast a PSA level rises than at whether or not your PSA level is above or below an absolute threshold, as has been the practice.

To make an informed decision, you'll need to thoroughly understand the debate, the pros and cons of the test, as well as your own risk factors for prostate cancer.

To start, let's review how the test works. The prostate normally secretes a small amount of PSA into the blood. Benign enlargement, inflammation, prostatitis, and cancer allow more PSA than normal to enter the bloodstream. The prostate cancer screening test simply analyzes your blood to see how much PSA it contains. The PSA is measured in nanograms (one-billionth of a gram) per milliliter (one-thousandth of a liter).

Traditionally, anything less than 4 ng/ml was considered normal, and above that level doctors recommended a biopsy to check for cancer. But this is not a hard-and-fast rule. In fact, it's a threshold research has thrown into question. Different doctors interpret these results differently. Over the years, some have used an age-adjusted scale that raises the threshold for biopsy as a man ages because his PSA levels increase naturally. Others have pushed for reducing the cut-off to as low as 2.5 ng/ml to pick up more cancers. Recent data from the Prostate Cancer Prevention Trial indicated three surprising findings: 1) 25 percent of men with a normal digital rectal examination (DRE) and PSA of less than 4.0 have prostate cancer on biopsy; 2) 15 percent of these men have high-grade cancers that are potentially lethal; and 3) there is no PSA below which the risk of having cancer is zero, with even 6 percent of men with a PSA score of less than 0.5 having cancer. These findings have further questioned whether a "normal" PSA value exists. Researchers have challenged the medical community to give up the idea of a "normal" PSA level below which a biopsy isn't needed. Instead, they have found that aggressive and potentially dangerous prostate cancers occur at PSA levels well below the traditional cut-off of 4 ng/ml.

Generally, though, a PSA level between 4 and 10 indicates a 25 percent chance that you have prostate cancer, according to the American Cancer Society. Some recent studies hint that the risk may be a little higher in this group, but more research is needed to prove that. If your level is over 10, you have a 67 percent chance of having prostate cancer, and the risk of cancer increases as the level continues to climb.

Be sure to alert your doctor if you have any conditions that can elevate PSA levels. These include prostatitis, urinary tract infections, prostate enlargement, and any procedures performed on the prostate such as surgery. In older men, ejaculation can cause the prostate to transiently leak more PSA into the blood. Be aware, too, that certain drugs, like finasteride and dutasteride and possibly some supplements, can lower your PSA levels. This may turn out to be a good thing. One recent study has found that finasteride appears to increase the sensitivity of the PSA test and may actually cause it to pick up more cancers (see Box 4-2).

Moreover, the PSA test is imprecise because both benign and malignant tissue can cause elevations in the blood. About one-fifth of men with cancer don't have PSA levels elevated enough to cause concern. Two-thirds of men with elevated PSA levels do not have cancer. That's why screening guidelines call for the PSA test to be used in conjunction with a digital rectal exam. In such an exam, a doctor will insert a gloved finger into the rectum to feel the prostate through the rectal wall. In this manner, he can tell if there are any lumps or other abnormalities that might indicate cancer. By itself, this exam isn't sufficient to screen for cancer because the doctor won't be able to feel a cancer that is still in an early, microscopic stage. But the exam does find cancers that PSA tests miss because some men with prostate cancer have low PSA levels. Some studies have estimated that digital rectal exams would catch somewhere between 10 and 17 percent of cancers that would not be picked up by a PSA test alone. If you decide to be screened, you should ask for both tests, because at this time that's the method least likely to miss a cancer.

NEW FINDING

Box 4-2: Finasteride aids PSA screening

A recent study found that finasteride appeared to improve the sensitivity of the PSA screening test, leading to the detection of more prostate cancers.

The study was published in the *Journal of the National Cancer Institute* and looked back at the PSA test results of nearly 10,000 men enrolled in an earlier trial of finasteride. When the PSA screening test results for men on finasteride were compared to those of men on placebo, researchers found that those on finasteride were less likely to have their prostate cancer missed by the screening test. This was true at all levels of severity, from the lowest-graded cancers to the highest. Because of this effect, men taking finasteride should have a better chance of having a prostate cancer detected by a PSA test than men who don't take the drug.

Your doctor is also likely to consider the results of a number of other tests done at the same time as the PSA screening test that can help him decide whether a biopsy makes sense for your particular situation. PSA velocity, which measures the change in your PSA levels over time, is getting more attention. Two studies found that an increase in PSA levels of more than 2 ng/ml in the year before a cancer diagnosis greatly increased the risk of death from prostate cancer. This was true despite the fact that the patients in the studies were treated with either radiation or surgery, and it was even true for some men who appeared to have low-risk cancers. However, more research is needed to confirm these results. Some doctors have suggested that older men with a rise in their PSA velocity of more than 0.5 in a year get a biopsy. But research is needed to determine if that threshold is really an indication of trouble.

In the first study, published in the *Journal of the American Medical Association* in July 2005, men whose cancers appeared to be low-risk had a 19 percent chance of death within seven years if their PSA velocity was greater than 2 ng/ml in a year. None of the men in the study with PSA velocities less than 2 ng/ml died in the seven-year term of the research. This study looked at 358 men treated with external beam radiation therapy. Researchers suggested men with PSA velocities greater than 2 undergo hormone therapy in combination with radiation because it may improve their chances of survival. Another study, published in the *New England Journal of Medicine* in July 2004, looked at 1,095 men who underwent surgery to remove the prostate after a cancer diagnosis. It found that men whose PSA increased by more than two points in the year before diagnosis had a significantly higher risk of death from prostate cancer than those whose PSA increased by less than two points. Up to 28 percent of men with PSA velocities above 2 died within seven years after surgery. But they were unable to determine exactly how much higher their risk was. The researchers suggested that aggressive treatment may be warranted for those men with higher PSA velocities.

Your doctor may also consider a free-PSA test, which measures whether the PSA in the blood is floating free on its own or is attached to a protein molecule. Benign conditions tend to produce more free-PSA while cancer tends to produce the attached form. By measuring the ratio of free to attached PSA, doctors get another hint about the cause of an elevated PSA level. PSA density tests, which require a prostate ultrasound to calculate, look at PSA levels in relation to the size of your prostate. Along with these tests, a number of other tests to help improve the reliability of PSA screening are under study.

The debate

Supporters of screening argue that the test can detect prostate cancers in an early, treatable stage about 80 percent of the time. In general, cancer that is caught before it spreads is easier to treat, and your chances of surviving the disease go up. In the case of prostate cancer, you have a nearly 100 percent chance of being cured if it is caught when confined to the gland. However, of men whose cancer has spread beyond the prostate, only about a third will survive for more than five years, according to the American Cancer Society. The overall 5-year survival rate has increased from 67 percent to 98 percent in the past 20 years. Supporters of screening argue that is evidence that screening saves lives. Recent research indicates that PSA screening cuts your risk of prostate cancer spreading by more than a third.

But opponents say a closer look at the numbers provides plenty of reasons for caution. The vast majority of cancers caught by screening are slow-growing and may never threaten the life of the patient, so treating these cancers exposes men to unnecessary side effects. The survival rate began increasing before prostate screening became common, indicating that the cause may have more to do with improved treatments than with screening. Also, survival rates have improved across the board—even in areas where PSA screening is not common. Studies that looked at whether screening saves lives so far have had mixed results, and there is little evidence to date that it helps. For example, one study compared Medicare beneficiaries in Seattle, where PSA screening was common, and in Connecticut, where it was not. It found no significant difference in the death rate from prostate cancer in the two areas after 11 years. But a similar study in Austria did find a small but significant reduction in prostate cancer deaths in areas where screening was widespread. Another study found that screening did reduce the death rate from prostate cancer. But it did not extend the lives of the men who were screened because they tended to die of another cause in about the same amount of time. All of that is cause for caution, screening opponents argue. To find out if screening really does save lives, men who are screened and those who aren't must be followed and compared for many years in a clinical trial. Those studies are underway, but the results will not be available for several more years.

Another reason that declining death rates may not mean that lives are being saved is that screening itself may distort the numbers. Prostate screening has created a big increase in the number of cancers diagnosed, and they are usually picked up at an early stage. But only six percent of prostate cancers eventually spread and become deadly; the vast majority grow very slowly and may never threaten the life of the patient, particularly older patients. So screening may cause doctors to treat many cancers that never would have killed the patient. However, those people are counted in the cancer statistics as survivors when in previous years their cancers—and successful outcomes—would have been ignored. That alone would cause death rates to look as if they're falling without actually saving any lives.

This is where it gets sticky. Opponents of screening say that it subjects thousands of men every year to needless biopsies and other medical procedures which carry the risk of bleeding and infection, and cause unnecessary anxiety. In addition, they argue that screening leads to treatment of a lot of cancers that aren't life-threatening at all. This subjects men to the risk of treatments that can cause impotence and incontinence, seriously eroding their quality of life without actually extending their lives.

Proponents argue that may be worth the risk because screening offers the chance to catch the minority of patients who have aggressive cancers before it's too late, so that at least for some men, it can be a life-saver. It's often difficult for doctors to distinguish which cancers are non-threatening and which will spread, so screening and treating all cancers is the only way to save that minority of men who have life-threatening disease, they argue. They point to studies that suggest the benefits of early treatment may take as long as 15 to 20 years to show up, indicating that studies have failed to find a clear-cut benefit to screening because they haven't followed men for enough years. Also, recent research has indicated that screening does pick up some dangerous cancers early.

The majority of men whose prostate cancers were found through PSA screening have clinically significant cancers, according to a June

2004 study in the *Archives of Internal Medicine.* The study looked at 977 patients with cancers that couldn't be picked up by a physical exam but which were referred for further testing after PSA screening. None had cancer that had spread, but the researchers evaluated their risk and determined that 61.5 percent had clinically significant disease based on biopsies and other tests. About 13 percent had high-risk tumors, and another 4.6 percent had intermediate-risk tumors. The study defined a clinically significant cancer as one that caused a 50 percent lifetime risk of dying from prostate cancer or of having a recurrence of cancer after surgery. This was estimated by determining a patient's normal life expectancy and estimating his annual risk. So an older man with a short life expectancy would need a high-risk cancer to meet that threshold. But a young man with many years ahead of him would face the same risk even if he had a slow-growing cancer because it would have time to develop into something dangerous. However, you should know that researchers have found contradictory evidence on the threat of slow-growing cancers eventually turning deadly. The most recent findings indicate that many slow-growing cancers remain stable even after 15 years and are unlikely to threaten lives. The real problem is that there are currently no diagnostic, pathologic, or radiographic tests that can tell what the biologic potential of an individual tumor is.

Medical organizations are split in their recommendations. The American Cancer Society and the American Urological Association recommend that screening be offered every year after age 50, and earlier for those at high risk. Most U.S. government agencies—the National Cancer Institute, the Centers for Disease Control and Prevention, and the U.S. Preventive Services Task Force—do not recommend widespread screening, though they agree it should be offered to those who want it. Other organizations, like the American Medical Association, recommend doctors inform their patients about the pros and cons of screening and leave the decision to them. This debate will continue until studies have shown definitively whether screening saves lives.

Researchers are also determining whether a change in screening methodology might make the process more practical, by sparing men who don't need treatment and catching more men with aggressive cancers whose lives can be saved by early intervention. One study indicated this could be accomplished by repeat PSA tests before

Box 4-3: Do all men need an annual PSA test?

A new study has found that men with very low PSA readings can probably safely skip some annual screenings, while those with levels above 1.5 ng/ml should not.

The study, published in the *Archives of Internal Medicine* in September 2005, looked at 5,855 men who were given annual PSA tests and biopsied if their PSA level was above 3. The men were followed for more than seven years and over that time cancer was detected at the following rates:

PSA score (ng/mL)	Percentage of men who had cancer detected
0 to 0.49	0.0
0.50 to 0.99	0.9
1.00 to 1.49	4.7
1.50 to 1.99	12.3
2.00 to 2.49	21.4
2.50 to 2.99	25.2
3.00 to 3.99	33.3
4.00 to 6.99	38.9
7.00 to 9.99	50.0
10.00 and above	76.8

Of the men with PSA levels below 1, no cases of cancer were detected in three years of follow-up. Researchers concluded that men with these low-PSA levels did not need to be screened every year and could safely be allowed to have a PSA test every three years.

But at the same time, they found that men with PSA levels between 1.5 and 2.9 had a risk of between 12 and 25 percent of being diagnosed with cancer in the next eight years. So they recommended close surveillance and annual screening of these men.

proceeding to other medical procedures such as biopsy. Another study indicated that screening at an earlier age, but only every couple of years, might pick up more-aggressive cancers while sparing the less-aggressive ones. A new finding indicates that men with very low PSA levels do not need to be screened every year, but those with levels above 1.5 ng/ml should be (see Box 4-3). Some researchers are looking for other chemicals or antibodies to prostate cancer that might give a clearer indication of whether a cancer is dangerous or not. Another possibility is genetic testing that could pinpoint those at highest risk who need the most screening, and also identify which men routinely have high PSA levels, absent cancer, so they can be spared unnecessary biopsies.

Making your decision

When you are discussing PSA screening with your doctor, you should consider your risk factors for prostate cancer. The biggest risk factor is simply age. About 96 percent of all prostate cancers occur in men over 55 years old. The risk climbs as men age—that's why most medical organizations recommend screening only begin when a man is in his 50s. But the cancers diagnosed in older men are much more likely to be slow-growing and non-threatening. So some doctors recommend that screening stop at about age 75, because any cancer that's present is likely to grow so slowly that it won't shorten the patient's life. He may well end up dying of something else before the cancer causes symptoms. Others believe screening ought to start on men in their 40s because these men have long lives ahead of them, during which the cancer could grow, and cause them to die.

One study found that higher PSA levels in young men, even when they are less than 4 ng/ml, may indicate a greater risk of developing prostate cancer later in life. The study, published in the September 2005 *Journal of Urology*, looked at 325 men who had blood drawn at an average age of 34 as part of a completely separate study. The researchers went back and measured those PSA levels. They found that even though the PSA levels were below the normal threshold of 4 ng/ml, the higher the PSA levels were at a young age, the more likely the men were to develop prostate cancer later. Black men with the highest levels of PSA were 4.4 times more likely to develop prostate cancer than those with the lowest youthful PSA levels. White men with the highest PSA levels were 3.5 times more likely to develop prostate cancer. Researchers suggested that youthful PSA levels could be used to target those men with the highest risk so they can get regular screening.

Race is another risk factor. African-Americans are twice as likely to die of prostate cancer as whites or Hispanics, while Asians, Pacific Islanders and Native Americans are at a lower risk, according to the National Cancer Institute.

Here's a look at your risk of developing prostate cancer by age and ethnicity:

Risk during the next 15 years (per 1,000 men)

Race/Ethnicity	At age 50	At age 65
All	2	16
African American	5	34
American Indian & Alaska Native	2	9
Asian & Pacific Islanders	1	7
Hispanic	1	12
White	2	14

Chart from: www.cdc.gov.

You may also be at increased risk if you have a family history of prostate cancer, particularly in a father or brother. There's also some evidence that you are at increased risk if you are overweight or eat a very fatty diet.

Once you have considered your particular risks, you may also want to think about your temperament and whether and how you would want to treat a cancer if it were found.

Some men decide they want screening because they want to do everything they can to reduce their risk of dying of prostate cancer. They are willing to risk treating a harmless cancer unnecessarily, even with the risk of side effects, in order to protect themselves.

Others fear the risk of impotence and incontinence more than the relatively small chance of dying of prostate cancer, which is only about three percent for the general population. So they choose not to be screened, sometimes because they don't want to know if they have a cancer that might worry them into a treatment decision they don't want to face. ■

5. UNDERSTANDING PROSTATE CANCER

Prostate cancer has gone public in the last decade. With alarming regularity, some public figure announces he is contending with the disease, from John Kerry and Rudy Giuliani to rock singer Johnny Ramone, who died of the disease in September 2004. A public-awareness campaign designed to promote prostate cancer screening has pounded home the alarming fact that prostate cancer is the second-most-deadly cancer for men after lung cancer. This is true, but it's important to keep fears about prostate cancer in perspective. While prostate cancer is extremely common—the American Cancer Society expects about 234,460 men to be diagnosed in 2006—it is one of the most survivable cancers. About one in six men will be diagnosed with prostate cancer sometime during their lifetime, but only one in 34 men will die of it. However, for a small group of men, prostate cancer can be deadly: about six percent of men are diagnosed when the cancer has spread throughout the body, and only 34 percent of them survive for five years. Still, heart disease is 10 times more likely to claim your life.

In short, you are far more likely to die with prostate cancer than from it. It can take 10 to 20 years for a prostate cancer, diagnosed when it is still small and contained in the gland, to grow serious enough to cause symptoms or threaten a man's life. Because the cancer strikes mostly older men at the end of their natural life expectancy, many simply die from something else long before the cancer requires treatment.

It's not always possible to determine whether you have an aggressive or passive form of the disease. Doctors have developed several scales that help them predict the odds for your prognosis, but they have limitations, and many cancers fall into a murky gray area. Because of this uncertainty, plus uncertainty about the relative benefits of many treatment options, figuring out what to do about prostate cancer can be an agonizing decision. It helps to understand what's known about the cancer itself, which we will cover in this chapter, as well as the pros and cons of various treatments, which we will present in the next chapter.

Prostate cancer basics

Nearly all prostate cancers begin in the glandular cells of the prostate, which produce the fluids that go into semen. They may begin changing years before a cancer is detected, as genes in the cells slowly mutate, producing abnormal cells that eventually evolve into cancer. As cancer cells mutate into more deadly forms they accumulate more abnormalities, start to grow out of control, cluster into tumors, and may eventually begin to invade other parts of the body.

No one is entirely sure what causes prostate cancer. It may well be a mix of factors, including genetic susceptibility and environmental factors such as diet or chemicals that cause genetic mutations. Researchers have identified at least 10 inherited genetic mutations that seem to increase the risk that a man will get prostate cancer. More suspect genes are being researched. Having one of these genetic defects does not mean a person will absolutely get prostate cancer but it does make it more likely. This is probably why some families have a history of prostate cancer. (For example, some families have a history of breast cancer in women caused by defects in the BRCA1 and BRCA2 genes. Their male relatives may also be at a slightly increased risk of developing prostate cancer, but this is thought to account for an extremely small percentage of cases.) Recently DeCode Genetics announced that it had identified a gene that raises the risk of prostate cancer by about 60 percent and may account for about 8 percent of all cases. The gene is about twice as common in African-Americans, who are at increased risk for the disease, as it is in men of European descent. More research is needed, but the scientists hope to develop a test that will make it easier for doctors to determine which cancers are dangerous and need aggressive treatment. Overall, only five to 10 percent of prostate cancer cases are estimated to arise from these inherited genetic susceptibilities, leaving researchers to puzzle over the cause for the vast majority of cases.

Lifestyle and environment are the chief suspects. Prostate cancer is far more common in Western Europe and North America than in other parts of the world. It is particularly low in Asia, but when Asians immigrate to the United States their risk increases. This leads researchers to suspect that diet may play a large role, but that remains unproven. Several studies have linked an increased risk of prostate cancer to diets high in fat, particularly from red meat. Other studies have found that vegetables may offer some protection from prostate cancer. Some, but not all studies, indicate that those who eat a lot of tomatoes, which contain an antioxidant called lycopene, may have a reduced risk of the disease. Eating a lot of cruciferous vegetables like broccoli, Brussels sprouts, or cauliflower may also reduce risk. One new study has found that pomegranate juice may slow the progression of prostate cancer, though more research is needed (see Box 5-1). Another intriguing recent study found that an ultra-low-fat diet, in combination with exercise and other lifestyle changes, might benefit prostate cancer patients. But all these studies are small and have limitations—they do not provide concrete medical evidence that these factors can protect you from prostate cancer.

In one study, a radical vegetarian diet—combined with a complete lifestyle overhaul—reduced PSA levels and researchers speculated it might prevent prostate cancer from worsening, according to recent research. The study, conducted by Dean Ornish, MD, an expert on the links between diet and heart disease who is known for his diet books, was published in the September 2005 issue of the *Journal of Urology*. It looked at 93 men with slow-growing prostate cancers who were assigned to either conventional therapy or Ornish's strict program of diet, exercise, and stress management. The Ornish program requires a vegetarian diet with less than 10 percent of calories from fat, regular exercise, and stress-management classes like yoga. Most of the men in the conventional treatment group opted to have their cancer monitored closely by doctors but did not opt for treatment. But six ended up getting treatment during the study because their cancer started to progress. After one year, patients on the Ornish program saw their PSA levels decline by four percent, while men in the comparison group saw their PSA levels rise by six percent. None of the patients on the Ornish program needed conventional treatment because their cancers did not progress. While the study provides a hint that a diet and lifestyle approach might benefit prostate cancer patients, there are some large caveats. The study followed a small number of men who had low-grade cancers with a good prognosis. It only followed the men for a year, and prostate cancer can take more than 10 years to turn dangerous. These very small changes in PSA level may not mean much at all—the only way to determine the value of diet and lifestyle changes is to see if they make a concrete difference in prostate cancer death rates over the long haul.

There is increasing evidence that being overweight increases your risk of prostate cancer. Recent studies have linked prostate cancer, as well as many other major cancers, to obesity and determined that the more a man weighs the more likely he is to die of prostate cancer. But not all studies have confirmed this link. One study conducted by the American Cancer Society found that obese men were 27 percent more likely to die of prostate cancer than normal-weight men. The more obese a man is, the higher his risk of being diagnosed with a more dangerous form of prostate cancer, another study found. That study, published in July 2005 in *Urology*, looked at 787 men who underwent prostate biopsy at a VA Medical Center in California. Obese men, defined as having a body mass index (BMI) over 35, were more likely to be diagnosed with prostate cancer than normal-weight men. The BMI is the ratio of height to weight. The higher a man's BMI, the more likely he was to be diagnosed with a high-grade, more aggressive cancer. In addition, new research has found that obesity raises the risk of prostate cancer recurrence after treatment, and that obese men are more likely to have their cancer detected at a later stage (see Box 5-2).

Researchers are also looking at the possibility that inflammation of the prostate, whether from a virus, prostatitis, a sexually transmitted disease, or some other cause, may be linked to prostate cancer. They believe that inflammation may damage cells, causing the mutations that eventually lead to cancer. But this research is in the early stages, and the question is far from settled.

Other potential causes of prostate cancer under study include chemicals, radiation, and high levels of male hormones like testosterone. The testosterone issue is causing growing alarm among researchers because many men are receiving testosterone replacement therapy to treat a variety of ailments that have been linked to lowered testosterone levels, from depression to loss of muscle and bone mass. The rate of such supplementation has increased 500 percent since 1993, and there is growing concern that, like hormone replacement therapy for women, the therapy is gaining popularity before sufficient research has been done on the risks. To date, there is no definitive

NEW FINDING
Box 5-2: Prostate cancer may be more dangerous in obese men

Some recent studies have found that prostate cancer may be more dangerous in obese men than in men at a healthy weight.

One study, published in the journal *Urology* in November 2005, found that obese men were more likely to have a recurrence of their cancer after treatment. The study followed more than 2,100 patients who had their prostates surgically removed for about two years. It found that the most obese men were 69 percent more likely to have a recurrence of their cancer, as measured by a climbing PSA level after the surgery. The more overweight a man was, the more likely his cancer returned after treatment.

Another study found that obese men were more likely to have larger prostates at the time of diagnosis with prostate cancer—a hint that their cancer was probably detected later. The study, published in the *Journal of Urology* in February 2006, looked at more than 1,400 men whose prostates were surgically removed. It found that in men under 63, the average prostate weight of men at a healthy weight was 33.8 grams compared to 41.4 grams for men who were obese.

Because it is harder to detect cancer in a larger prostate, researchers suggested that obese men were more likely to have their cancer detected at a later stage when it is more difficult to treat and more dangerous to the patient.

However, not all research has confirmed these findings so more studies will be needed to determine if obesity does indeed increase your risk of aggressive prostate cancer.

evidence that testosterone supplementation causes prostate cancer. But there have been scattered reports in the medical literature of men with normal prostate exams developing prostate cancer after starting to take testosterone therapy. Some studies have shown that men with higher testosterone levels are at a greater risk for prostate cancer and that testosterone can make prostate cancer grow more aggressively. In fact, one way of treating late-stage prostate cancer is to reduce testosterone levels to slow the cancer down.

Because the causes of prostate cancer are unknown, there is no sure way to prevent it. Most of the risk factors for prostate cancer—race, age, and family history—can't be changed. But researchers are looking at a number of factors that may contribute. The National Cancer Institute is conducting a major trial of the antioxidants selenium and vitamin E to see whether they might reduce the risk of prostate cancer, but it will be several years before there are results. The drug finasteride, commonly used to treat prostate enlargement, was recently found to prevent some prostate cancers but also to slightly increase the risk of aggressive prostate cancers. Most urologists do not recommend it as a preventive strategy at this time. Recent but very preliminary research has hinted that some drugs may help prevent prostate cancer, but these findings need to be confirmed by more research before they can be used as a preventive therapy. Among the candidates are the cholesterol-lowering drugs known as statins, a combination of vitamin D and non-steroidal anti-inflammatory drugs, the 5-alpha reductase inhibitor dutasteride (Avodart), and the breast cancer drug toremifene (Acapodene).

A number of diets that are low in fat or high in soy, which is thought to possibly tamp down the hormones that stimulate cancer, are under study.

Though there is not enough scientific evidence to prove such interventions can really prevent prostate cancer, there are a number of healthy lifestyle choices you can make that may help and will probably boost your health overall.

- **Adopt a low-fat, high-fiber diet** like the one in the federal government's food guide pyramid (www.MyPyramid.gov). Both high-fat diets and obesity have been linked to increased risk of prostate cancer in a number of studies.

- **Eat more vegetables**, particularly tomatoes, which contain lycopene, an antioxidant that some studies have found may reduce your risk of prostate cancer. Other potential sources of lycopene or other potentially helpful antioxidants include grapefruit, watermelon, garlic, broccoli, cabbage, and arugula.
- **Exercise regularly.** This can help control your weight, which may be a risk factor. It may also help you reduce some urinary symptoms. Some studies, though far from proven, indicate that exercise may help lower your overall cancer risk.

Testing and diagnosis

Unfortunately, early prostate cancer often produces no symptoms, which is why it sometimes isn't caught before it has spread, greatly reducing the chances of survival. When symptoms do appear, they mimic those of benign prostate conditions like prostate enlargement. But today, many cases of prostate cancer are caught early with widespread screening.

Though prostate cancer symptoms are rare, if you experience these symptoms you should see your doctor:

- Loss of appetite and weight
- Difficulty urinating
- Bone pain
- Pain in the lower back, hips, or lower pelvic area
- Pain during urination or ejaculation
- A weakened stream of urine, dribbling, leaking or interrupted urine stream
- Frequent need to urinate, particularly at night
- Blood in the urine
- The feeling that your bladder isn't empty.

If you do have symptoms or an elevated PSA test, your doctor will want to start by ruling out other causes for the problem. He may order a urine test to check for infection and will almost certainly do a physical exam to see if he can feel any lumps, growth, or changes in your prostate.

Your doctor may also order other tests, such as a free-PSA test or PSA velocity, which can give him additional information in order to judge your risk of cancer. He may request a transrectal ultrasound, a

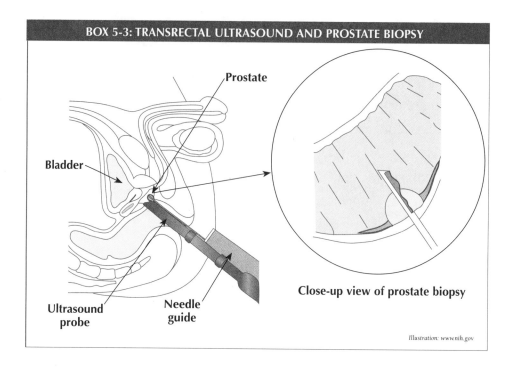

BOX 5-3: TRANSRECTAL ULTRASOUND AND PROSTATE BIOPSY

Prostate

Bladder

Close-up view of prostate biopsy

Ultrasound probe

Needle guide

Illustration: www.nih.gov

procedure in which a probe is inserted into your rectum and sound waves are emitted to take a picture of your prostate. This can tell the doctor if there are any abnormalities that might indicate cancer, although most prostate cancers are invisible on ultrasound.

But if these tests indicate cause for concern, the only way to tell for sure whether or not you have cancer is through a biopsy. A tiny sample of prostate tissue will be removed and studied under a microscope to determine if cancer is present (see Box 5-3).

This is usually done with a procedure called a core needle biopsy. An ultrasound probe and a spring-loaded needle are inserted in the rectum. The ultrasound is used to guide the doctor to all areas of the prostate to ensure a thorough sampling. Then the needle, which moves in a fraction of a second to prevent pain, is inserted into the prostate through the wall of the rectum to remove a tiny sample of tissue. The doctor may take a dozen or more of these samples from different areas of the prostate.

The whole procedure takes only about 15 minutes and can be done in your doctor's office. The procedure is usually done under local anesthesia, so you should feel little discomfort; bear in mind that the procedure does carry a small risk of bleeding and infection.

Sometimes a biopsy will find no signs of cancer, despite other tests that indicate a high likelihood that you have it. In that case, your doctor may have to repeat the procedure. This happens because the prostate contains many tiny tumors, invisible on ultrasound, spread in areas of the prostate that may be missed by random sampling. For this reason, even if your biopsy indicates you don't have cancer, you should return to the doctor for periodic testing to make sure that nothing is amiss.

Once the biopsy has been done, the samples will be sent to a laboratory; a doctor will analyze it to see if you have cancer, and if you do, estimate how aggressive it is. If you do have cancer, your doctor may want to perform a variety of other tests to determine how aggressive your cancer is and whether it has spread to other parts of your body.

The most common tests you may need include:

- **A bone scan,** to see if cancer has spread to your bones.
- **A chest X-ray** to see if cancer has spread to your lungs, or elsewhere in the chest.
- **A computerized tomography, or CT scan,** to identify abnormalities in your lymph nodes or other organs in the pelvis. This test can't tell you whether those problems are due to cancer, however, so you may need further tests to clarify its findings.
- **A magnetic resonance imaging (MRI)** test can also take pictures of the body, giving doctors an indication about whether cancer has spread to the seminal vesicles.
- If doctors suspect your cancer has spread, you may need a **lymph node biopsy.** Since many cancers are caught early due to PSA screening this isn't as common a procedure as it used to be. The biopsy may be performed as part of the surgery to remove your prostate, with a needle, or in a separate surgery. A lab will analyze a sample of the nodes to look for signs of cancer.

Grading and staging your cancer

Once your doctors have gathered as much information as they need, they will assess how dangerous your cancer is. This is done by grading and staging your cancer. To grade a cancer, doctors look at how closely it resembles normal tissue. Low-grade cancers are the least aggressive and look most like normal tissues. High-grade cancers are the most abnormal and are more likely to grow fast and spread aggressively. To stage a cancer, doctors look at how far the cancer has already spread. Again, an early stage means that the cancer is likely to be contained within the prostate and a higher stage means it has spread outside of the prostate. Though this system can be confusing, understanding it will help you assess your risks and make an informed decision about treatment.

One caveat: different doctors and hospitals may use different terminology or different staging and grading systems. You may have to question your doctor to fully understand the implications of the stage and grade he has assigned to your cancer.

A Gleason score is the most common form of grading prostate cancers. It will be determined after your biopsy, based on a doctor's examination of the tissue under a microscope. The doctor will look for irregular cells under the microscope, then assign a score to the two most common types of cells. The scores are based on a scale of one to five, with one being the least-aggressive and five the most-aggressive cancer. The scores of both types are then added to get the final score on a scale of two to 10.

A Gleason score of two to four is considered a low-risk cancer, meaning the odds are low that it will spread beyond the prostate in the next five to 10 years. A score of five to seven is considered a medium-risk cancer, and a score of eight to 10 is considered a high-risk cancer. Many pathologists will not actually diagnose a cancer unless the Gleason score is at least 6.

The Gleason score is important because it can help predict the future course of your cancer, even if it has been caught early and does not appear to be very serious yet. Your Gleason score will be considered along with the stage of your cancer, to help determine which treatments are best for you. In general, the higher your stage of cancer, the higher the threat to your life and the more treatment you may need. Also, you should know that some recent research has found that those whose PSA scores climbed more than 2 ng/ml in a year may have an increased risk of aggressive cancer—even when their Gleason scores were low. For more information, see chapter 4.

There are several different methods for staging prostate cancers, but the one most commonly used in the United States is the staging system of the American Joint Committee on Cancer, called the TNM system. This system looks at tumor size, whether the cancer has spread to the nearby lymph nodes, and whether it has spread to distant parts of the body. Different doctors may use slightly different versions of the system, so you may want to discuss your precise TNM score with your doctor. But the TNM scores break down into four basic categories that form the basis for treatment decisions and are based on how advanced your cancer is. Here are the four basic categories:

- **Stage I** indicates cancer that is completely confined to the prostate and is still in a microscopic stage that can't be felt by your doctor.

- **Stage II** means your cancer is contained within the prostate and has not spread, but it may be big enough to be felt by your doctor when he does a physical exam, as a lump or unfamiliar texture. It may involve more of the prostate gland. Or you may have a medium to high Gleason score, indicating a somewhat more aggressive cancer that has not yet spread.

- **Stage III** means your cancer has begun to spread beyond your prostate, but it hasn't gotten very far. It may have just invaded the seminal vesicles or other tissue immediately surrounding the prostate, but it has not reached the lymph nodes or other parts of the body.

- **Stage IV** means your cancer is widespread. It may have invaded your bladder, rectum or pelvis, or it has been found in your lymph nodes or other parts of the body. ■

6. PROSTATE CANCER TREATMENT

As scary as any cancer diagnosis is, your first impulse may be to rush into treatment. Don't do it. Take a moment to catch your breath and carefully think through your options. Unless you have an aggressive form of the disease there is little risk to waiting a few weeks or even months, because prostate cancer is usually slow-growing. In fact, one new study suggests you could wait up to two years before undergoing surgery (see Box 6-1). Take your time and gather all the information you need to think through your decision. It won't be an easy one. The main options for early prostate cancer are surgery, radiation, and active surveillance—skipping treatment completely, but having the condition monitored closely by a doctor so that there is time to act should it become dangerous. Hormone therapy and chemotherapy are also an option for some patients. So far, research isn't clear cut about which options work best for which men. Longer studies are needed to settle the question. To complicate the picture, treatments continue to evolve and improve—but that often means that existing research is outdated because it was done on older therapies.

Our understanding of the risks of the various treatments is also evolving. In the short run, different treatments seem to carry different risks of impotence, incontinence, and other side effects, but in the long run recent

NEW FINDING

Box 6-1: Delaying prostate cancer surgery is safe

A new study has found that delaying surgery and undergoing active surveillance does not lead to a higher incidence of non-curable cancer.

The study, published in the *Journal of the National Cancer Institute* in March 2006, looked at men with small, low-grade tumors. Researchers compared 38 men in an active surveillance program that delayed surgery an average of 26.5 months to 150 patients with similar characteristics who had immediate surgery. Then they checked to see how many of the men developed a non-curable cancer—one that carried less than a 75 percent chance of remaining disease free for 10 years.

After adjusting for age and PSA density, they found no statistically significant difference between the two groups. So they concluded that active surveillance for up to two years is safe and does not increase the risk of developing a non-curable cancer. A large, NCI-sponsored randomized trial called START, designed to compare active surveillance to immediate treatment, is now underway in the U.S. and Canada.

research suggests this tends to equalize. In general, it appears that the side effects of surgery, mostly impotence and incontinence, occur quickly but that with radiation sexual function tends to decline over the years. But again, because treatments are evolving, often in ways intended to minimize side effects, there hasn't been enough time to conduct long-term studies that would help judge the most current options.

You'll want to consider the pros and cons of each treatment, relative to your own situation and how aggressive and advanced your cancer is. As you're thinking about your decision, here are a few important points to consider:

- **Start with the stage and grade of your cancer.** Talk with your doctor to fully understand how aggressive the cancer is that you're dealing with. Your doctor should give you a sense of how well the three options should work for your situation and what the risk of side effects will be for you.

- **Consider your age and health.** A young man in his 50s with many decades ahead of him may want to treat a cancer aggressively to maximize his chances of surviving as long as possible. But a low-grade cancer in a man in his 70s is likely to be slow-growing and may not have time to progress to a dangerous stage before he reaches the end of his life from some other cause. This is particularly true if he is in poor health, which can also make treatment more risky. High-grade cancers can still be life-threatening even in men who are 70 or older and are generally treated.

- **Think about your quality of life after treatment.** Both radiation and surgery can cause impotence. Surgery can also cause incontinence, and radiation can cause other urinary and rectal symptoms. You may have to make some difficult and personal tradeoffs in the face of uncertainty about how different options will work. Some men choose to delay treatment or non-surgical options because they fear their sex life may be harmed. Others are more fearful of dying or of the anxiety of living with an untreated cancer and prefer surgery despite the risk of impotence.

- **Be sure you are getting balanced, impartial and complete information.** Research has found that many doctors advocate the treatment option they are most familiar with or that they perform themselves. That may or may not be the right choice for you. You may want to get a second opinion from a doctor who specializes in a different kind of treatment. For example, you may want to visit a radiation therapist if your first doctor is a surgeon. Be sure that you feel comfortable discussing all your options with your doctors and that they take the time to answer all of your questions. You should also do your own research on each of the options so you are fully informed and not just relying on your doctor's opinion. After all, you are the one who will have to live with this decision. Recent research indicates that many men newly diagnosed with prostate cancer rush into treatment decisions based on anecdotes and a faulty understanding of their options (see Box 6-2). So take your time and be thorough.

- **Think about how well you will tolerate uncertainty and repeated doctor's visits to deal with your cancer.** If you are considering active surveillance, will it worry you to know that you have untreated cancer inside you? Will you be rigorous about returning to the doctor for repeated testing? Or would you feel better with aggressive treatment?

With these issues in mind, here is a look at the pros and cons of various treatment options.

Surgery

Surgery to completely remove the prostate is one of the most common treatments for prostate cancer. Today, most of these procedures are done in a way that attempts to spare the nerves that control your bladder and erections, reducing, but not eliminating, the risk of incontinence and impotence.

The most common form of surgery is retropubic radical prostatectomy, in which doctors remove the prostate through an incision or a scope in your abdomen. This incision, which runs from your navel to the pubic bone, allows surgeons ample access. It gives them room to maneuver around your nerves to reduce complications and also permits them to remove your lymph nodes for testing.

Sometimes, the surgeon will access the prostate perineally, through an incision made between your anus and scrotum. This reduces bleeding, and if you are overweight, recovery time. But it makes it difficult to spare the nerves and offers no access to the lymph nodes.

Both forms of surgery are difficult and complicated procedures, and they can take up to four hours to perform. You may need to stay in the hospital for about three days and wear a catheter to drain urine for one to two weeks. Up to 10 percent of patients have complications such as bleeding, infection or heart problems. There is a very small risk of death from surgery, which is greater for older men or those in poor health.

Two relatively new forms of minimally invasive prostate surgery are becoming more common and may have certain benefits. Laparoscopic surgery does not require the large incision that open prostatectomy does and therefore may cause less scarring and pain, and facilitate faster recovery. Early research indicates that it is about equivalent to open surgery in terms of removing cancer and preventing recurrence as well as in the rates of complications like impotence and incontinence. However, because the procedure is still relatively new there hasn't been enough long-term, published research to be sure of this. Some unpublished data that has been presented to other physicians publicly indicates that rates of incontinence after laparoscopic surgery may be significantly worse than in open prostatectomy

In laparoscopic surgery, carbon dioxide gas is pumped into the abdomen to lift the abdominal wall so the surgeon can see better. Five small incisions are made to insert surgical instruments and a small camera that allows the doctor to see what he's doing. Then the surgeon simply uses the camera to guide him as he removes your prostate.

Sometimes laparoscopic surgery is performed with a robot, which gives the surgeon a better view of what's going on inside your body. In robotic surgery, incisions are made to allow three robotic arms to do the actual work of the surgery. One contains a high-resolution camera and the other two perform the surgery itself. The surgeon actually sits several feet away at a computer console and controls the robotic arms via a joystick and foot pedals. The robotic arms eliminate hand tremors and provide extremely fine control for precision movements inside the body.

Like laparoscopic surgery, robotic surgery seems to allow men faster recovery rates with fewer immediate surgical complications. The rate of success, as well as of impotence and incontinence appears to be about the same.

But if you are considering either minimally invasive surgery, you should be very careful in selecting a surgeon. These are new and very complicated procedures and they take significant training and skill to perform well. Be sure to ask how many of these procedures your surgeon has performed. A recent comparison of open, laparascopic and robotic surgeries can be seen in Box 6-3.

Risks

Most men lose control of their ability to urinate after surgery, and the problem may last for months. The vast majority of men gradually improve over time, but about 10 percent continue to have occasional problems with leaking after coughing or other stress. One percent or less have a more severe long-term problem that can be fixed by placement of an artificial sphincter. Men who have perineal surgery may also experience a higher likelihood of fecal soiling on their underwear.

Nerve-sparing surgery has reduced the risk of impotence, but many will lose some degree of sexual function. Estimates of how widespread impotence is vary hugely—from about 20 to 70 percent—according to different studies. This may be because different men face different risks. If you are older, were already having trouble maintaining an erection before surgery, or have a more widespread cancer, you are more likely to suffer impotence after surgery. Research also shows that you are more likely to have complications if your operation is performed by a less-experienced surgeon or in a hospital that does not handle many prostate surgeries. If you decide on surgery, you should look for a surgeon who specializes in the procedure.

Sometimes, even after the prostate is removed, the cancer reappears. This occurs when the cancer has spread beyond the prostate, though that is not always detectable before or during surgery. If your PSA level begins to climb after surgery, your doctor may suggest salvage radiation therapy. However, research studies on the benefits of this have produced a wide range of results—from 17 to 64 percent of men seemed to benefit from the procedure. Patients with the most aggressive cancers were least likely to benefit. More research is needed to determine the real benefits and risks of salvage radiation therapy. Recent research in the *Journal of the National Cancer Institute* has focused on developing models to predict whose cancer will return and is a good candidate for salvage radiation. This procedure also raises your risk of side effects, so you will need to carefully weigh the risks and benefits of this procedure with your doctor, should it become an issue. Some doctors also use hormone therapy for patients whose PSA levels rise after surgery, but the evidence for this is very mixed, and the treatment has not yet been proven to help.

Benefits

For many men, prostate cancer surgery provides peace of mind because it removes the source of the cancer. Very often, no further treatment is needed. Men whose cancer has not spread beyond the prostate have a 90 percent chance of surviving and being cancer free at least 10 years after surgery. Research to date hasn't determined whether surgery is more effective than radiation. But a recent study did find that surgery was more likely than active surveillance to prevent spread of the disease and death from prostate cancer over a 10-year period. Prostate cancer patients who had surgery were 44 percent less likely to die of the disease in the first 10 years after surgery than men who opted for active surveillance, researchers found.

The study, published in May 2005 in the *New England Journal of Medicine*, updated previous shorter-term results by adding three more years of follow-up to the study. Men who had surgery were 40 percent less likely to have their cancer spread throughout the body and 67 percent less likely to have it progress locally. However, though these percentages are large, they affected relatively few men. The study followed 695 men randomly assigned to surgery or active surveillance. Of the men who had surgery, 30 of 347, or 8.6 percent, died of prostate cancer in the first 10 years of the study. In the active surveillance group, 50 of 348 men, or 14.4 percent, died of prostate cancer. The researchers noted that surgery seemed to benefit younger men more than older men. Men over 65 may not have benefited from surgery at all—though they cautioned that their study wasn't designed to answer this particular point and more research is needed to determine which patients are most likely to benefit from surgery.

The study is continuing, and researchers expect the benefits of surgery to grow as men are followed for even longer periods of time. However, they also cautioned that the study began before the age of widespread screening, which has resulted in many cancers being caught much earlier. This could mean that the benefit of surgery may be less definitive in men who come in for treatment at a much earlier stage. Or it could mean that smaller tumors are easier to treat and result in fewer complications from surgery. They suggested more research is needed on the value of surgery in the age of widespread screening.

Radiation

As far as we know, radiation is about as effective as surgery to prevent cancer from spreading over a 10-year period. A review of existing research on the issue in the *Canadian Journal of Urology* found that there wasn't enough clear evidence to say which option was best. The American Urological Association has updated its prostate cancer guidelines to reflect this lack of evidence, saying that either surgery or radiation are acceptable options.

There are two forms of radiation, and each carries different potential risks. The standard treatment, called external beam radiation, uses powerful X-rays to attack the cancer. It can also damage nearby tissue. To minimize this risk, you will go through a number of careful body scans that help radiologists pinpoint the exact margins of the prostate. New computer technology can create exquisitely accurate maps and help doctors precisely focus the radiation beams so higher doses can be delivered with less damage to nearby structures. This technique may reduce side effects and work better than older technology, but the technology is new so long-term research is needed to confirm such potential benefit.

However, recent research indicates that men who receive high-dose external beam radiation are less likely to have their cancer recur than men who get a conventional dose. The study, published in September 2005 in the *Journal of the American Medical Association*, followed 393 patients who were given either high-dose or conventional-dose radiation therapy. After five years, 80.4 percent of the patients given high-dose radiation were free of the rising PSA level that would indicate a possible recurrence of their cancers. Of those given a conventional dose, 61.4 percent also did not have increases in their PSA level. The high-dose patients were 49 percent less likely to have a recurrence, but they were also twice as likely to suffer side effects like serious urinary and rectal problems. Such problems affected two percent of high-dose patients and about one percent of conventional-dose patients. However, more research is needed to determine whether high-dose radiation will actually save more lives than conventional-dose radiation. This study found no significant difference in overall survival rates between the two groups.

External beam radiation treatments only take about 15 minutes each day but can be time-consuming, as you will have to go to the hospital every day for about two months. You will be strapped into place to be sure you are in the correct position so the beam doesn't accidentally damage tissue it's not meant to hit. You may also be given custom-built lead shields to protect vital organs. The treatment is not painful, but side effects will accumulate as the therapy goes on. Most men will have urinary problems like burning and increased frequency during treatment. You may also have diarrhea, bleeding from the rectum, and painful or difficult bowel movements. Most of these problems will be temporary but they may subside gradually over several months. Radiation also can cause fatigue and loss of appetite, which should subside in the months after treatment is completed.

A newer and increasingly popular form of radiation therapy is radioactive seed implants. This treatment works best for small to medium-size cancers and may reduce the rectal symptoms of radiation, but it causes more urinary problems. This form of radiation therapy, known as brachytherapy, may not be a good option for men with more aggressive forms of prostate cancer, some research indicates. Doctors implant small radioactive pellets into your prostate that can deliver a higher dose of radiation than the external beam procedure. Using an ultrasound guided needle, doctors will inject up to 200 pellets, depending on the size and location of the cancer. This is about an hour-long procedure done on an outpatient basis.

In the most common procedure, the pellets, about the size of a grain of rice, remain inside you forever. They emit a form of radiation that travels only a few millimeters so that the radiation is unlikely to extend beyond your prostate, thus hopefully reducing complications. However, because they're inside the prostate and closer to the urethra they cause urinary problems in nearly all men. Some patients need a catheter at times to help them urinate during the six months that the radiation lasts. These urinary symptoms tend to be more severe than in external beam radiation. Some doctors use higher-dose pellets that are left inside the prostate only temporarily.

The radiation in the pellets can take up to a year to be completely exhausted, depending on what material is used. The technology is so new that long-term study results aren't available yet to prove whether it works as well as external beam radiation or surgery. But at least one study has found that at eight years of follow-up, seed and beam radiation worked equally well.

Also, research indicates that combining radiation therapy with hormone therapy improves the survival rate of patients with aggressive cancers that have spread a little beyond the prostate but not yet spread throughout the body. The study, published in August 2004 in the *Journal of the American Medical Association*, looked at 206 men with aggressive cancers that had spread beyond the prostate but not widely throughout the body. They were assigned to either external beam radiation or radiation plus six months of drugs that block the male hormones that can fuel the growth of prostate cancer. The five-year survival rate of those with the combination therapy was 88 percent, compared to 78 percent for those who had radiation alone. Patients who had the combination therapy were also less likely to see their disease progress to a stage where they required subsequent hormone therapy to extend their lives. A previous study had found a survival benefit for combining three years of hormone therapy with radiation, but this study found that a shorter dose, which lowers the risk of side effects, was also beneficial. Because this study looked only at patients with aggressive cancer, meaning a Gleason score of 7 or above and cancer that had already started to spread beyond the prostate, it's not known if combination therapy makes sense for other patients. More research is needed to determine whether patients with less-aggressive, earlier-stage cancers might benefit and whether it would be worth the risk of added side effects. Hormone therapy carries its own risks, such as impotence. More research is needed to determine which patients are most likely to benefit from this combination therapy and to determine the best dose.

Risks

Radiation carries somewhat different risks of side effects than surgery. Urinary and bowel problems are more common in radiation. But incontinence is less common in radiation than in surgery. Impotence is less of a risk immediately after treatment but tends to increase slowly over the years, and it may reach as high as 50 percent or more. Some long-term research indicates the risk of sexual problems is as high in radiation as in surgery after five or more years.

One study found that five years after treatment, patients who received external beam radiation were just as likely as patients who had surgery to experience sexual problems because their sexual function continued to decline. They were less likely than surgery patients to have incontinence problems. The study, published in September 2004 in the *Journal of the National Cancer Institute*, followed 1,187 men who had either radiation therapy or surgery. It found that after five years the level of overall sexual function in men who underwent radiation had declined to the same levels as those of men who had surgery. Men who received radiation therapy had only a four percent rate of incontinence, while 14 to 16 percent of surgical patients reported problems. Radiation patients were more likely than surgical patients to report bowel problems. However, researchers note that these patients were treated in

1994 and 1995, and improvements in surgical and radiation techniques, plus the advent of brachytherapy, may lead to different results in patients being treated now.

Urinary problems due to radiation therapy are usually temporary, but they can go on for months, both during the therapy itself and as they gradually subside after therapy. Rectal problems from external beam radiation can also last for months, and a tiny fraction of men require surgery to correct these complications.

Radiation doesn't cause immediate impotence the way surgery can, but it does create problems that gradually arise in the months after treatment. This is because radiation can damage the nerves that control the penis and the arteries that carry blood to it. Many men will experience at least some trouble getting or maintaining an erection. External beam radiation is thought to cause impotence in about half of all patients. The newer seed therapy can cause impotence in 30 to 50 percent of patients, and some researchers are beginning to question whether it preserves more sexual function than external beam radiation. More long-term research is needed to clarify this issue. As with surgery, you are more likely to retain sexual function if you had it before therapy and if you are young.

There is also a risk that the cancer will recur. In addition, seed therapy is not effective for tumors just outside the prostate and may not work as well as other treatments for aggressive and larger tumors.

Benefits

Radiation carries less risk of death (not that the risk of death with surgery is high) and other serious complications because there is no surgery or anesthesia involved. Though the side effects are unpleasant, undergoing radiation can be less debilitating and less painful than having to recover from a major operation. External beam radiation can be used to treat cancers that have spread into the pelvis and cannot be removed surgically. It can also be used in men with advanced disease that isn't curable, to help shrink tumors and reduce pain. There is less risk of permanent urinary problems than with surgery. But for those undergoing external beam radiation there is a risk of permanent bowel problems.

Active surveillance

For some men, the best treatment may be no treatment at all. This is an option because more and more men are discovering prostate cancer at an extremely early stage thanks to the widespread use of prostate screening. In active surveillance, formerly known as watchful waiting, you won't be given any treatment unless your doctor detects signs that the cancer is growing more aggressive. But you will have to return to the doctor regularly for blood tests, rectal exams, and biopsies to keep close tabs on the disease. You will also have to pay close attention to any symptoms you may have.

This is an option for those who have a cancer that is confined to the prostate and have a low-to-medium Gleason score. It is most often offered as an option to older men or those who are in poor health because it completely avoids the risks and side effects of treatment. Most of these men can live normally with their cancer and may die of something else long before it becomes a problem. But active surveillance can be an option for younger men who want to avoid the side effects of treatment or postpone it as long as possible. However, the evidence on the risk of this strategy for younger men is contradictory.

Men with low-grade prostate cancers have a minimal risk of dying even after 20 years without treatment, making active surveillance a viable option for them, one study has found. The research, published in May 2004 in the *Journal of the American Medical Association*, contradicts a smaller study that indicated prostate cancer death rates accelerate after 15 years without treatment. This study, which followed 767 men diagnosed with low-grade prostate cancer between 1971 and 1984, found that death rates actually declined after 15 years. It found that prostate cancer mortality was 33 per 1,000 person-years in the first 15 years of follow-up and that it dropped to 18 deaths per 1,000-person-years after 15 years. Both studies seem to agree that men with non-aggressive, slow-growing tumors rarely die from prostate cancer where men with aggressive tumors are more likely to die within 10 years of diagnosis, often despite getting aggressive treatment. One reason for the contradiction may be that the studies followed different populations of men and used different methods to determine how aggressive their cancers were. More importantly, both studies followed men who were diagnosed long before PSA screening became common. Today's prostate cancer patients are usually picked up earlier in the progress of the disease, and their long-term survival may be even longer as a result. A new study published in the *Journal of the National Cancer Institute* in March 2006 looked at the issue in a different way. It found that men who had surgery immediately had the same chance of developing a non-curable cancer as those who waited up to two years. Thus, there was little risk to waiting in the short term (see Box 6-1, page 48).

However, long-term studies will need to be done on current prostate cancer patients before we will have clear and definitive evidence about the risks of active surveillance.

Risks

With active surveillance, you are taking a chance that the cancer will grow into something dangerous. You must be vigilant about returning to the doctor for all necessary tests. You may be delaying treatment until you are older, when it is riskier and the chance of side effects is greater. In rare cases, a slow-growing cancer may speed up, and you could be caught short with a cancer that can no longer be cured. Also, by delaying treatment you may allow a cancer to grow to a size where it begins to cause urinary and other symptoms. You may worry about your fate, knowing you have cancer that isn't being treated. A new study found that about half of men who opt for watchful waiting abandon it within two years, not because their cancer worsens, but because they fear it will (see Box 6-4).

Benefits

You will avoid the risk of impotence and incontinence that comes with treatment. You also stand a very good chance of never developing

NEW FINDING

Box 6-4: Questions raised about active surveillance

A review of research on active surveillance has raised questions about the best way to monitor men who opt to delay treatment.

The research, published in the *Journal of Urology* in August 2006, looked at five studies that included a total of more than 450 men with localized prostate cancer.

The men were monitored in many different ways including using PSA levels, digital rectal exams, additional biopsies and other tests like PSA velocity. The researchers could not determine which form of monitoring was best because of the limitations of the studies.

Up to half the men sought treatment within two years, even though most didn't show signs of disease progression—because of their anxiety that it might.

However, the researchers determined that because these men were at low risk, active surveillance was a viable option for them. More research is needed to figure out the best way to design such programs and the best way to monitor these men.

symptoms or requiring treatment. Even if your cancer grows, it's likely it will do so slowly. If it does grow, you may benefit from new, more-effective and less-risky treatments that may be developed in the future. Research has shown that for at least the first eight years, the life expectancy of men who choose this option appears to be no different than those who choose to treat their cancer aggressively.

Hormone therapy

This form of therapy was first used to treat men with advanced prostate cancer that can no longer be cured, and it has been shown to improve their quality of life. Hormone therapy can't kill the cancer, but it may extend your life, though the research on improvements in long-term survival is unclear. But today, hormone therapy is also used on many men whose cancer is less advanced—and the merits of that are being debated. One recent trial found that it improves survival when given in combination with radiation therapy to men whose cancer is aggressive and has started to spread beyond the prostate.

However, hormone therapy is often given to men whose cancer does not appear to have spread beyond the prostate but whose PSA levels start to climb after treatment. There isn't yet good evidence that this practice does in fact improve survival, according to a recent review of medical research on the topic published in the *Journal of the American Medical Association*. Since hormone therapy carries risks, the researchers cautioned that we don't yet know whether the potential benefits of hormone therapy in this situation outweigh the risks.

Hormone therapy is based on the premise that male sex hormones stimulate the growth of cancer cells. By blocking those hormones, it can slow the growth of cancer. But eventually the cancer will become resistant to this treatment and begin to grow again.

Sometimes hormone therapy is also used in men with less-advanced cancers because it can shrink tumors to a size that makes them easier to attack with surgery or radiation.

The most common form of hormone therapy is drug therapy. You may be given a combination of different drugs that can block the effect of testosterone. The most common of these drugs are leuprolide (Lupron, Eligard, Viadur or Trelstar) and goserelin (Zoladex) which must be injected every three to four months, though longer-acting formulas are available.

Another class of drugs prevents your body from using testosterone, thus preventing cancer cells from being affected by it. These antiandrogens drugs are taken daily, and include flutamide (Eulexin), bicalutamide (Casodex) and nilutamide (Nilandron).

Sometimes doctors will start and stop hormone therapy in an effort to delay the cancer from becoming resistant and to decrease side effects.

Another option in hormone therapy is surgical castration, because removing the testicles eliminates the main factory of testosterone in the body. The procedure can be done under a local anesthetic and does not require a hospital stay. The testicles are removed through a small incision in the scrotum, and for men who want it, they can be cosmetically replaced with a prosthesis. Surgery is irreversible, but drug therapy can be stopped at any time to reduce side effects. Drug therapy does cause additional risks over surgery, however, including heart problems and breast enlargement.

Risks

Hormone therapy does have serious side effects, although a new study indicates that some of the risks may be overstated (see Box 6-5). You may face a lowered libido, impotence, hot flashes, weight gain, breast

---

NEW FINDING

Box 6-5: Some risks of hormone therapy overstated

Androgen deprivation syndrome includes a range of symptoms such as depression, memory problems and fatigue and some researchers have linked it to hormone therapy for prostate cancer. But now a new study has found that while such problems are common in men on hormone therapy, they are probably not caused by the treatment.

The research, published in February 2006 in the *Archives of Internal Medicine*, looked at Medicare data on more than 100,000 men with and without prostate cancer. It found that of those who survived at least 5 years after a prostate cancer diagnosis, 31.3 percent developed at least one depressive, cognitive or constitutional symptom compared to only 23.7 percent of those who didn't get hormone therapy.

But then the researchers adjusted the data to account for the presences of other health problems, the severity of the cancer and age. They found that the difference between men on hormone therapy and those who weren't almost completely disappeared. So they concluded that the incidence of these symptoms is likely due to the fact that the men on hormone therapy were generally older and sicker.

Still, because these troubling symptoms affect nearly a third of men on hormone therapy, they advised doctors to do a better job of monitoring and treating patients for these problems.

tenderness, and a loss of strength due to a loss of muscle and bone mass. Some researchers have found evidence of depression and cognitive declines, but others have not. Hormone therapy for prostate cancer also increases the risk of fractures in older men because it reduces bone density, research has found. The study, published in January 2005 in the *New England Journal of Medicine*, looked at the medical records of more than 50,000 men with prostate cancer in a Medicare database. It found that 19.4 percent of patients who received hormone therapy had been treated for a fracture compared to 12.5 percent of those who didn't receive hormones. The drugs also may carry risks of breast enlargement, nausea, diarrhea, fatigue, and liver damage.

While hormones may delay death, they cannot prevent it. Eventually, advanced prostate cancer becomes resistant to hormone therapy, and it no longer works. There is also some evidence that hormones may increase the risk of heart problems.

Benefits

Hormone therapy can shrink tumors, thus reducing your symptoms and pain and possibly extending your life. Drugs can often lower your level of testosterone as effectively as castration, but they can be stopped at any time to eliminate the side effects they cause.

New approaches

Until recently, chemotherapy has not been used to treat prostate cancer, other than to control pain, because studies had failed to show that it prolonged survival. But that may change. A handful of studies have found that some chemotherapy regimens modestly extended the lives of patients with advanced prostate cancer, after hormone therapy failed. The FDA approved the chemotherapy drug docetaxel (Taxotere), commonly used to treat breast cancer, for use in advanced prostate cancer. Several studies are also looking at ways of combining docetaxel with other drugs to improve its benefits for patients. So far there is no evidence that chemotherapy is beneficial in earlier stages of prostate cancer before it has spread, but studies are underway to see if it might benefit patients.

One study found that the chemotherapy drug docetaxel combined with the steroid prednisone added an average of 2.5 months to the lives of patients, compared to a standard therapy designed to alleviate their symptoms but not extend their life. The study, published in October 2004 in the *New England Journal of Medicine*, looked at 1,006 patients with advanced prostate cancer that was no longer responding to hormone therapy. Until now, when prostate cancer became resistant to hormone therapy, there was nothing doctors could do to prolong life. Patients on the docetaxel regimen lived an average of 18.9 months, compared to an average of 16.5 months for those who were given a conventional chemotherapy regimen. Patients on the docetaxel regimen suffered more problems with lowered white blood cell counts, but their levels of infection and fatigue were similar to those on the conventional chemotherapy regimen. Based on this and a similar study which also demonstrated a survival advantage, chemotherapy is now considered the standard of care for men whose cancer has spread to their bones, when their cancer becomes resistant to hormones.

Other treatments are also being studied, though they have not yet been proven effective. Among them is cryosurgery, which uses liquid nitrogen to freeze and kill cancer cells in the prostate. It seems to reduce the urinary problems caused by surgery but does not have as much success with impotence. In fact, some studies have reported rates of sexual dysfunction after cryosurgery as high as 80 percent. It is still under study, so doctors cannot be sure how well it works in the long term.

Researchers are also studying cancer vaccines, which work by priming the body's immune system to kill off cancer cells, and angiogenesis inhibitors, drugs that work by cutting off the blood supply to growing tumors in hopes of starving them. The National Cancer Institute is combining cancer vaccines with hormone therapy, which appears to boost their effectiveness (see Box 6-6). Another avenue of research is targeted therapies, which can attack only cancer cells while sparing healthy cells, thus minimizing side effects.

Some men also consider using alternative therapies, such as herbal supplements, to combat their prostate cancer. If you decide to do that, you should discuss it with your doctors because some herbal supplements can interfere with the drugs or other therapy you are taking. There is no supplement on the market that has been adequately studied for use against prostate cancer so there is no evidence that any of them work.

Managing side effects

Many men face impotence after treatment for prostate cancer, but these days there are more options than ever before to help you cope. Men who have prostate cancer surgery typically have an immediate loss of sexual function that gradually improves. But it can take 18 months or longer for sexual function to return, and it may not reach the same level as before surgery. Men who have radiation therapy, either external beam radiation or brachytherapy, typically don't face an immediate loss of sexual function but may gradually see their sexual function decline over the following years. How well you maintain sexual function after radiation or recover it after surgery depends on many factors, including your age, the quality of your erections before treatment, and your general health before treatment. Chronic health conditions like heart disease and diabetes, lifestyle factors like obesity and smoking, and the use of certain medications can all affect your sexual health after prostate cancer treatment.

Typically, the first line of treatment is medication. Sildenafil citrate (Viagra), tadalafil (Cialis) or vardenafil (Levitra) can all be used to treat impotence that results from cancer treatment. These drugs haven't been studied head to head for the treatment of erectile dysfunction from prostate cancer treatment, so it's not known which, if any, is most effective. Also, you must recover or maintain enough nerve function after surgery for these drugs to work. Functioning penile nerves produce nitric oxide, which normally relaxes certain muscles in the penis, allowing blood to flow in and causing an erection. These drugs work by enhancing the ability of nitric oxide to produce an erection—but some nitric oxide must be present in order for them to work. For this reason, they are far more effective on patients who've had nerve-sparing surgery than on those whose nerves were damaged during surgery. A report in the *Journal of the American Medical Association* estimated that erectile dysfunction drugs worked in about 70 to 80 percent of men who had nerve-sparing surgery but only in up to 15 percent of men who had non-nerve-sparing surgery.

Some doctors have looked at whether impotence after surgery could be prevented by administering sildenafil nightly in the months immediately following surgery in hopes that early sexual stimulation and blood flow in the penis might hasten the return of natural, unassisted erections. One small study seemed to find that it did, but the strategy, known as erection rehabilitation, remains unproved, and more research is needed to see if it works.

Though these medications can help many people, some cannot take them. If you've had a heart attack, stroke, or heart rhythm irregularities in the past six months, you should not take these medications. If you have heart disease and have been warned that sexual activity might be dangerous, you should not take these drugs. In addition, if you take nitrate drugs, like the heart medication nitroglycerin, you should avoid these medications because the combination can cause heart problems, seriously low blood pressure, and dizziness.

Recently, the FDA added a warning to the label of all these drugs because of reports that they led to sudden vision loss. The drugs have been linked to a condition called non-arteritic ischemic optic neuropathy, or NAION, which can suddenly cut the flow of blood to the optic nerve. It's not clear that the drugs cause this rare condition because NAION and erectile dysfunction share many of the same risk factors. But the FDA warns anyone taking these drugs to stop taking them immediately if they experience sudden vision loss or decreased vision in one or both eyes. Patients who've experienced sudden vision loss in the past, or who've been diagnosed with NAION in the past, should avoid these drugs.

There are some other options. Some men benefit from prostaglandin E1, a substance the body produces that can cause erections. This product can be injected into the penis a few minutes before intercourse or delivered in a suppository. Side effects include pain, dizziness and prolonged erection. Vacuum pumps and penile implants can also be used to create an erection. These options usually work for men who've had too much nerve damage to benefit from sildenafil. They can also be used in the period after surgery before natural erections have returned—with one big caveat. It's best to avoid any therapy that might interfere with recovery of spontaneous, natural erections. For this reason, penile implants are not a good idea.

Some men also find that counseling helps them deal with the sexual side effects of prostate cancer treatment.

If you are dealing with urinary incontinence, after prostate cancer treatment, don't let frustration or embarrassment prevent you from talking to your doctor about it. There are some options to help control your symptoms. Treatment will vary depending on what's causing your incontinence and how severe it is. Sometimes doctors can prescribe drugs to help control the problem. Sometimes surgery to install an artificial sphincter or other methods can help. Some men with stress incontinence learn to cope by wearing special pads or briefs that can absorb any leakage. ■

CONCLUSION

Despite the uncertainty and confusion surrounding prostate conditions and prostate cancer, there is reason for hope. Prostate cancer death rates are falling rapidly. The advent of widespread PSA screening has brought the disease into the spotlight. Over the next decade, the results of long-term research should provide answers to difficult questions about the effectiveness of available treatments, their side effects, and the benefits of screening.

New treatments are under study. These include new drugs, surgical procedures, and even vaccines. Research into the genetics of prostate cancer may lead to far more accurate screening tests and help doctors figure out which cancers are deadly and need treatment and which may safely be left alone. This could spare thousands of men unnecessary procedures. Scientists are also working to fine-tune the treatments already in hand, to make the most effective use of them.

But in the short run, all this could mean more confusion: If you are faced with a prostate condition, especially prostate cancer, you may be faced with an expanding number of treatment options without the clear-cut evidence you need to figure out which treatments are best for you.

The best thing you can do is stop, take a breath, make time to educate yourself and consider all your options carefully. Don't allow anyone to rush you into a decision you're uncomfortable with. Remember that modern medicine doesn't have all the answers yet and that you are the one who has to live with the consequences.

We hope this report has given you some tools to make you more comfortable asking those questions and making these very personal decisions. ■